Tammy LaBrake, CSW

How to Get Families More Involved in the Nursing Home: Four Programs That Work and Why

Pre-publication
REVIEWS,
COMMENTARIES,
EVALUATIONS . . .

"**R**esearch has dispelled the myth that family members abandon their loved ones to nursing homes. However, family and psychological dynamics as well as the social stigma against aging and nursing homes can create varying levels of discomfort in family members when visiting their relative.

Ms. LaBrake's book recognizes that the needs of family members are as diverse as the resident population and that, therefore, a variety of programs and approaches should be developed to promote family involvement. Her book provides practical and creative 'how-to' ideas and instructions on planning, implementing, and evaluating these services for family members."

Marion Shackford, MSW
Vice President, Residential Services, Rochester, NY

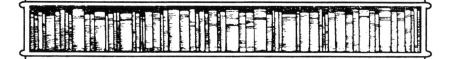

How to Get Families More Involved in the Nursing Home
Four Programs That Work and Why

THE HAWORTH PRESS
New, Recent, and Forthcoming Titles
of Related Interest

Leisure in Later Life, Second Edition, by Michael J. Leitner and Sarah F. Leitner

The Black Elderly: Satisfaction and Quality of Later Life by Marguerite Coke and James A. Twaite

Aging and God: Spiritual Pathways to Mental Health in Midlife and Later Years by Harold G. Koenig

Growing Up: Pastoral Nurture for the Later Years by Thomas B. Robb

A Guide to Psychological Practice in Geriatric Long-Term Care by Peter A. Lichtenberg

Quality of Life in Long-Term Care by Dorothy Coons and Nancy Mace

How to Get Families More Involved in the Nursing Home
Four Programs That Work and Why

Tammy LaBrake, CSW

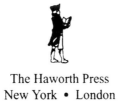

The Haworth Press
New York • London

The Haworth Press, Inc., 10 Alice Street, Binghamton, NY 13904-1580 USA

This book is not intended to represent the official position of the New York State Department of Health.

Paperback edition published in 1997.

Cover design by Monica L. Seifert.

Library of Congress Cataloging-in-Publication Data

LaBrake, Tammy.
  How to get families more involved in the nursing home : four programs that work and why / Tammy LaBrake.
     p.   cm.
  Includes bibliographical references and index.
  ISBN 0-7890-0205-1 (alk. paper)
  1. Nursing home patients. Family relationships. 2. Medical social work. 3. Social work with the aged. I. Title.
RA997.L33   1996
362.1′6–dc20   96-20595
                                                                                       CIP

CONTENTS

ABOUT THE AUTHOR

Tammy J. LaBrake, CSW, is Public Health Social Work Consultant for the New York State Department of Health in Troy. In this capacity, she regulates statutory requirements in nursing homes, conducts surveys of nursing homes, and identifies deficient practices where they exist. The previous Director of Social Work Services for the Delaware County Home and Infirmary in Delhi, New York, Ms. LaBrake is an expert on the organizational structures and operations of long-term care and regulatory systems. She is particularly interested in how the quality of physical environment and activity programs can empower residents and accommodate their needs and interests.

Preface

RECOGNIZING THE NEED

Regulations that govern residents' rights in nursing homes cite the Home as being responsible for the well-being of each resident. There are no statutes or rules about the responsibility of family in the nursing home, but the regulations reflect certain precepts about family involvement—one of them is that family programs should be offered to promote joint participation between the staff and family in sustaining the residents' well-being. The family is considered to be one of the best guarantees of the residents' well-being. Not only do family members keep the resident connected to the past, present, and future, but they also help prevent care from becoming wearisome and perfunctory. Family members help staff to assess residents' needs in relation to customary routines, lifetime patterns, and peculiar idiosyncrasies. In addition, the presence of the family in the nursing home lightens the institutional atmosphere.

FOUR PROGRAMS THAT WORK AND WHY

The development of a family program should be tailored to the unique needs of the nursing home and its family population. Offering more than one type of program is recommended to ensure reaching many different families. Some suggested programs follow.

Educational Workshops

Educational workshops offer an outlet to families for discussing aging-related topics and nursing home issues. These programs provide specific information, foster realistic expectations, and enhance staff/family communication. The family will learn to challenge misconceptions about aging and nursing homes.

Support Groups

Support groups provide families with a supportive setting in which to share questions and concerns. These programs offer a therapeutic environment for open lines of communication. The family often becomes emotionally adjusted to nursing home placement of a relative by participating in a support group.

Council Meetings

This type of program encourages families to play an active role in the operation of the nursing home. By participating in the decisions and events that affect the residents' lives, families help improve the residents' community and prevent services from deteriorating

Holiday Socials

Festive gatherings help build solidarity among family members. Families see that they are not alone and become increasingly comfortable with sharing nursing home experiences. This type of informal gathering encourages the attendance of otherwise reluctant families. Other family programs are also marketed at this type of event.

FULFILLING THE NEED

Family involvement is subject to progression or regression, depending on the amount of support and sanction given by the nursing home. By offering family programs, the nursing home sends a clear message that family involvement is important and welcomed. The overall outcome of family programming is a positive influence on the residents' well-being.

This book will give concrete suggestions on how to develop and implement the following family programs: Educational Workshops; support groups; Family Councils; and Holiday Socials. It is important to note that "family" refers to any relative or other person who visits or stays in contact with a resident of a nursing home.

Chapter 1

Educational Family Workshops

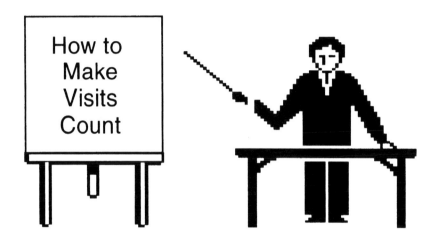

How to
Make
Visits
Count

PURPOSE OF THE FAMILY WORKSHOP

- To affirm the value of staff/family interactions
- To provide basic information about topics related to aging
- To give the family techniques to make visits productive and meaningful
- To foster realistic expectations regarding services and provision of care in the nursing home

HELPFUL HINTS ON GETTING STARTED

Table 1.1 projects the needs of a Family Workshop and provides suggestions for creating an educational setting.

SUGGESTED TOPICS FOR THE WORKSHOP

One way of tailoring the workshop to meet the unique needs of the nursing home and its family population is to assess the interests of the family population. A survey completed by families will provide information regarding common interests and willingness to participate in a Family Workshop. A sample of a survey has been included in the Appendix. Keep in mind that a survey indi-

TABLE 1.1. Workshop Characteristics

Considerations	Suggestions	Anticipated Outcome
physical setting	large conference room	good ventilation and space
seating arrangements	tables with chairs	easy note-taking
refreshments	cookies, fruit, beverages	energizing
# invited to workshop	total family population	15-33 percent response
method of invitation	mailing with RSVP	promotes reserving seats
duration of workshop	2 hours	allows ample time for Q&A
time/day of week	Sunday 2-4 p.m.	popular visiting day
season	late winter	nonactive time of the year
speakers	multidisciplinary	draw from expertise

cates interests, but not a commitment to actually attend a work-shop. To determine if family members will come to a workshop, you must invite them. Send families invitations to attend a Family Workshop and ask them to RSVP, which will show an interest as well as a commitment to attend. A sample of an invitation to attend a Family Workshop can be found in the Appendix.

The workshop should be well structured with emphasis on the topics that family members indicated they were interested in learning more about. The outcome of assessing their interests is likely to involve the following topics:

- Stress Associated with Aging
- Making Visits Count
- Enhancing Staff/Family Communication
- Understanding Medicare and Medicaid

Topic 1. Stress Associated with Aging

The purpose of this topic is to help family members realize their own attitudes about aging and to discover ways to acknowl-edge the negative and positive aspects of aging. This particular topic is meant to be an educational experience for workshop participants as they consider their own aging. Little information focuses on the resident during discussions of this topic.

What You Need to Begin

1. Four multicolored *index cards* with the following incom-plete sentences:

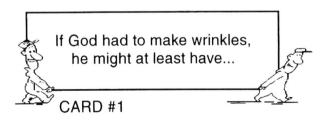

If God had to make wrinkles,
he might at least have...

CARD #1

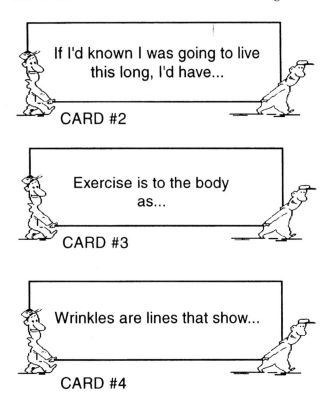

At the beginning of the session distribute the four cards to participants who are willing to read aloud to the group. Before beginning the session, ask all four people with a card to quietly read it to one other participant. This helps them feel more comfortable when they are later asked to read the card to everyone. They can also begin thinking about how to complete the sentence on the card.

2. An *overhead projector* to view transparency, "Stressors Associated with Aging."
3. Fine-point *markers* for the overhead.
4. A *poster* with an outline of the four topics to be discussed.
5. An *oven timer.*

In order to keep the workshop within two hours, time frames

are necessary. (The oven timer releases you from timekeeping duties and workshop participants are more at ease by knowing what time frames to expect.) Again, invoke participation by asking a family member to be responsible for the timer.

6. Three pieces of *scrap paper* and a pencil or pen for each participant.
7. *Name tags* for all attending.

Introductions

Encourage all participants, including staff members, to wear name tags. Before starting the workshop explain to the participants that you have invited several staff members to attend the workshop. Staff should be dispersed at different tables with family members. Formally introduce the staff by having them stand during introductions.

Members of the staff should include but not be limited to: the administrator; a physician assistant or nurse practitioner; a registered nurse, preferably the director of nursing; a dietitian; an occupational therapist and/or a physical therapist; a social worker, and a representative from the activities department. Then have each family member introduce him or herself. It is also helpful to have family members tell who their resident is and on which wing their resident resides.

Beginning the Topic

Topics related to aging can cause people discomfort. Because aging can be an uncomfortable subject, it is essential that families understand how their perceptions about aging influence the quality of their visits in the nursing home. As families become aware of their own fears and misconceptions about aging, they will become more comfortable during their visits. To begin this topic, ask the workshop participant who has card #1 to read it aloud:

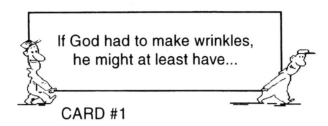

CARD #1

The purpose of these cards is not to spend an inordinate amount of time discussing the card, but rather to keep the discussion focused and light. Ask participants to complete the sentence from card #1. For example, "If God had to make wrinkles . . . why didn't he put them on the bottom of our feet!"

Your next opening statement should address the discomfort that discussing aging can cause. You could say, "Talking about getting old is not a very popular topic." Begin a more in-depth conversation by asking some or all of the following questions:

- How many of you feel you are getting old? How many of you *want* to get old?
- How many of you feel that visiting a nursing home causes you to think about your own aging?
- In what way does this influence the quality of your visits?
- If folks have come to terms with their own aging, will they be more comfortable visiting a nursing home?
- If they have not come to terms with their own aging, are they likely to avoid spending much time in a nursing home?
- So, how does one come to terms with aging and the stress related to aging?

Share with the group that one way to come to terms with one's own aging is to prepare for the stress that can be associated with the aging process.

Identifying the Stressors That Are Associated with Aging

Participants should already be divided into small groups with five to eight people at a table. Tell each table to assign a "leader" who will keep notes. Each staff member sitting at a table should offer support and help facilitate discussion when necessary. Instruct the participants at each table to discuss among themselves some of the stress they believe to be associated with aging. Set the timer and allow five minutes for discussion.

While discussion is taking place, you should give some direction to the participants by listing on an overhead transparency different categories of stress such as: SOCIAL STRESS, FINANCIAL STRESS, PSYCHOLOGICAL STRESS, STRESS OF BODILY CHANGES. To enhance visual effect, use different colored markers for each category.

When the timer sounds, remove the transparency of stress categories from the overhead and replace it with a more detailed description of the kinds of stress that can be associated with aging. It is easier and less time consuming to have a description of stressors associated with aging already printed and ready to use on an overhead transparency. Consult the Appendix for a list of age-related stressors. Ask each "leader" to report the kinds of stress discussed at his or her table, and place a check mark on the transparency next to each type of stress identified. Any types of stress not listed on the transparency can be added with a marker.

Now that the participants have talked about stressors associated with the aging process, ask if any of them have thought about ways to cope. While they are thinking, have the holder of card #2 read it aloud and ask the participants to complete the sentence:

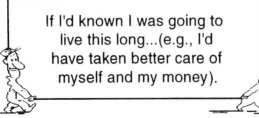

If I'd known I was going to live this long...(e.g., I'd have taken better care of myself and my money).

CARD #2

Ask the holder of card #3 to read it aloud:

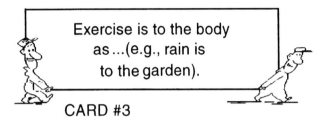

Exercise is to the body
as...(e.g., rain is
to the garden).

CARD #3

Ask participants how a 100-year-old person might complete this sentence, "One of the best things about getting old is . . ." Inquire if participants know an older person who lives life to the fullest every moment of the day. (It is a golden moment when a participant names his or her own resident.) Do they know what helped that older person discover such energy and love for life? Display a poster on which the following is written: "Youth is for learning; adulthood is for service; old age is for self-discovery." Then ask participants to share: (1) what they learned as a child; (2) what service they have provided as an adult; and (3) what they hope to discover about themselves when they are elderly.

Ask the workshop participant who has card #4 to read it aloud:

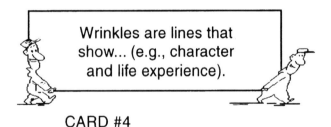

Wrinkles are lines that
show... (e.g., character
and life experience).

CARD #4

Tell participants to complete this sentence on a scrap piece of paper: "Today I will remember that despite my age I . . ."

While family members are doing this, assemble staff members at the front of the room to prepare for a brief question and answer (Q&A) period. Before starting the Q&A period, ask if any participants would like to share what they wrote on their scrap piece of paper. Then invite family members to ask staff any questions they might still have about identifying and coping with the different kinds of stress associated with aging. Questions on "how to make visits count" should be withheld until later when that topic is discussed. Any questions concerning finances should be withheld as well. Allow five to ten minutes for Q&A. (Remember to set the timer.)

Staff members should come to the workshop prepared to offer their own recommendations on how to cope with stress. For example, the dietitian might present information on healthy diet habits. The occupational therapist or physical therapist might give exercise tips. The social worker might discuss ways to cope with the psychological stress associated with aging. The physician assistant might address questions about age-related diseases and how to avoid or minimize the risk of such diseases. The physician assistant might also address whether or not certain diseases are inherited. Prior to the workshop, meet with staff and ask them to bring literature and/or suggestions on how to cope with aging.

The participants should be prompted to ask questions about their own concerns about aging, but it is important to note that during this Q&A period, family members will be likely to express concerns about the care their resident is receiving. For example, a family member might say, "My mother says she is not getting any exercise; is that true?" Naturally, a staff member will address this concern in a way that fosters realistic expectations regarding services and provision of care in the nursing home. It may be necessary to suggest a private meeting with a family member who is clearly distressed and is unable to resolve his or her issue in this type of format.

Since staff members and family were sitting side-by-side at the tables, family members may not ask very many questions at this time because staff members have already answered questions at the tables. After questions have been answered, have staff members return to the tables for the next topic.

Topic 2. Making Visits Count

Families who have residents who are withdrawn, confused, and/or constantly asking to go home often get frustrated during visits. The purpose of this topic is to discuss techniques that will make visiting more enjoyable.

What You Need to Begin

1. A *handout* of "Tips on How to Make Visits Count" (See the Appendix.)
2. An *overhead projector* to view the handout
3. A *shoebox* for every participant (Remind staff to bring shoeboxes in one week before the workshop.)
4. A *script* for role-playing printed on index cards for staff members (Rehearsing a few days before the workshop is recommended.)

Beginning the Topic

Ask participants if their resident is ever forgetful, confused, or disoriented. Tell participants that it is not uncommon for families to get frustrated by this. It is hard to know what to say or do when a resident no longer recognizes family members. It can also be difficult to visit a resident who is always asking to go home or who is, on the other hand, withdrawn and noncommunicative. Explain that the purpose of this topic is to introduce families to techniques for making visits productive and meaningful. A representative from the social work and/or activities department should present information that incorporates tips on making visits count. These tips should be distributed in the form of a handout and reviewed by using an overhead projector. Tips to include for making visits count can be found in the Appendix. To help participants incorporate some of the information, use the following activities:

Activity 1. Making a Shoebox of Memories. To demonstrate how to make a shoebox of memories, have one or two staff members come prepared to share his or her own shoebox of memories. For display purposes, the shoeboxes staff share should be covered with contact paper. During this demonstration it would be helpful if a staff member shares a musical tape that triggers particular memories. A bouncy musical piece would serve as a good example of what to include in a memory box, while also energizing the participants who have been sitting for awhile at the workshop. Play this tune and invite the workshop participants to stand and stretch or even dance!

After being rejuvenated by the music, each participant is given a shoebox and asked to think about what he or she would put inside that could trigger memories for his or her resident. Family members should consider their resident's religion, musical interests, ethnic background, occupation, favorite leisure-time activity, traveling experiences, family life, and daily routine prior to the need for nursing home placement. Have each participant write his or her ideas on a piece of paper and place it inside the box. Staff should help the participants think of memories to put in the shoebox that will include things to touch, smell, and hear. Urge each participant to fill the box at home with the actual items and bring it on the next visit.

Activity 2. Role-Playing. Explain to workshop participants that they will now view a role-play situation between a "resident" and a "family member." Staff who will be role-playing should have had an opportunity to rehearse prior to the day of the workshop. If staff are uncomfortable doing this "live," show a videotape of the role-play instead. The purpose of the role-play will be to show an effective way to address the questions of a resident with dementia. For example, the following script demonstrates two ways a resident with dementia can be responded to after he or she has stated "I want to go home." After each role play ask the "resident" the questions that are outlined in the script.

Script for Role-Play

Part I

Resident: I want to go home now . . . can you take me?

  Visitor: This is your home now. Your house is sold.

Resident: I want to go home! Do you have a car?

  Visitor: You had to give the house up . . . you couldn't live there alone . . . remember?

Suggested Question: Ask the "resident" how it feels to hear that his house is sold . . . to be told that he had to leave home because he could no longer take care of himself.

Part II

Resident: I want to go home now . . . can you take me?

  Visitor: Where is your home?

Resident: It's just down the road. . . . Do you have a car?

  Visitor: What do you want to do when you get home?

Resident: I've got to make dinner for Joe.

  Visitor: What do you want to make for dinner?

Resident: Beef stew.

  Visitor: Well, we need to call Joe and tell him to pick up some of the food at the store.

Resident: Joe won't be home right now.

  Visitor: Well then, let's write a list of things we need at the store so we won't forget what we need.

Suggested Question: Ask the "resident" if she is thinking of the house, the food, or Joe right now? Ask how it felt to talk about cooking dinner for Joe. The "resident" will probably say that she felt validated. Ask family members why they think this approach was more effective in calming the "resident."

Topic 3. Enhancing Staff/Family Communication

Heightening the family's awareness of the many barriers that can hinder staff/family communication is a fundamental step in enhancing communication. Once barriers are identified, ways to break through them are presented.

What You Need to Begin

1. A *list* of key personnel and department heads with respective telephone extensions.
2. *Index cards* for questions family members may not want to say out loud.
3. A blank *"wish list"* for family members to give to administration.

Staff should come prepared to talk about tips on how staff and family should communicate with each other.

To Begin the Topic

Have staff return to the front of the room to present ideas on successful ways for staff and family to communicate. The following should be emphasized during this discussion:

1. Rewarding interactions between staff and family encourages future interactions. A barrier that can hinder staff/family interactions is when a conversation has been more costly than rewarding. This happens when one person is ignored, criticized, or just misunderstood. A rewarding interaction occurs when both parties feel heard. Both parties do not necessarily need to agree but they need to feel understood, which often involves a compromise.
2. Explain that the most important part of communication is body language and tone of voice, not the actual words that

are used. A barrier that can hinder staff/family interaction is when staff members appear hurried and rush through the corridors. Another barrier is created when voices are raised during discussions. No matter how angry one might become, it is best to talk with a calm, nonthreatening tone of voice.

3. Family members should know that their visits, questions, and input on how to care for their resident are welcomed by the staff. A barrier that can hinder staff/family interaction is when families feel unwanted or awkward. Ask participants for advice on how to make sure families feel wanted and comfortable during their visits.

4. Discuss different forum options to allow for regular staff/family communication such as:

   a. General family meetings on a regular basis
   b. Family support groups to help deal with feelings
   c. Special holiday activities
   d. Annual care-planning meetings
   e. Annual policy-making meetings
   f. Family socials during holidays
   g. Educational workshops for families
   h. Panel discussions with department heads

After staff members have shared the above ideas on how to overcome barriers that can hinder staff/family interactions, have staff members return to the tables where the family members are seated. Then ask family members for examples of positive interactions they have had when talking with the staff in the past. It is important to note that a family member is likely to mention a negative experience at this time. If this happens ask the participants, including staff members, what could have made the interaction more positive or rewarding. Keep the focus on the quality of the interaction and not the actual problem that the family member was discussing at the time. If necessary, the problem can always be discussed after the workshop has ended.

To end this topic ask participants to communicate with the administrator by completing the following "wish list":

Dear Administrator:
If I were granted three wishes, here is what I would wish:
For my resident, I wish: _____
For the staff, I wish: _____
For the nursing home, I wish:_____

Topic 4. Understanding Medicare and Medicaid

This is a topic that reaches out to families who otherwise might not attend the workshop. A representative from the County Department of Social Services and a reimbursement specialist from the nursing home are recommended to present information on this topic.

What You Need to Begin

1. *Handouts* or literature relevant to Medicare and Medicaid.
2. A suggested *outline* for guest speakers to follow.

   a. Medicaid and Medicare overview
   b. Eligibility and enrollment
   c. Services covered and not covered
   d. Co-payments and deductibles
   e. Prior-approval procedures
   f. Recertification
   g. Fair hearings and appeals
   h. Advantages of keeping other insurances
   i. Long-term care insurance

Be aware that when finances are involved, the discussion can become heated. For example, a family member might charge,

"When my mother came to this nursing home, she had to sign her house over to Medicaid. Have you ever tried explaining that to your mother? Well, guess who gets blamed!" When questions such as this one are raised out of anger, the family member should be advised that his or her concerns could be more effectively addressed privately, with a DSS worker. His or her feelings can be validated, but the purpose of this topic is meant to be informative.

Some family members will attend the workshop primarily to learn about Medicaid and Medicare. This is especially true for family members who are concerned that their resident will soon need to apply for Medicaid. Questions related to applying for Medicaid are usually straight-forward and this topic takes no more than 20 to 30 minutes.

EVALUATION FOR THE WORKSHOP

Prior to dismissing the workshop, urge the participants to complete an evaluation form. This will provide feedback that assesses effectiveness and offers suggestions on ways to improve the next workshop and future topics. A sample evaluation form for this workshop, as well as for the programs presented in the following chapters, can be found in the Appendix.

SAYING GOODBYE

At the conclusion of the Family Workshop, inform participants of the next scheduled family event. Stand at the door as family members exit, thank each one for attending, and be certain to shake hands. It is important to give each family member special attention as he or she leaves, taking note of his or her comments, and recognizing his or her involvement in the nursing home. Saying goodbye is an important part of ending all of the programs presented in the following chapters.

This chapter described in detail how to use an educational workshop to enhance communications between family and staff. Also presented were ways to help families feel more comfortable visiting their resident.

The techniques presented in the next chapter will help you to create a support group in which families can learn how to manage the problems and/or feelings of having a loved one in a nursing home.

Chapter 2

Family Support Groups

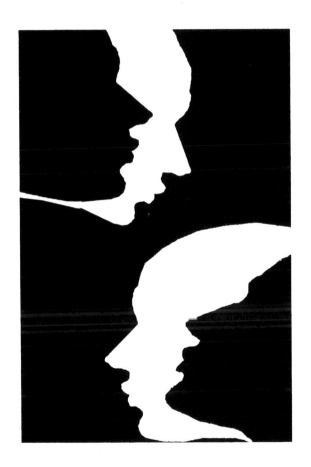

PURPOSE OF THE FAMILY SUPPORT GROUP

- To create a supportive environment for family members to air their concerns and feelings about placing a loved one in a nursing home
- To build family solidarity by providing an opportunity for family members to connect and realize areas of common ground
- To help families understand the various stages of adjustment to nursing home placement
- To provide an educational opportunity for families to learn how to manage the problems or feelings of dealing with a loved one in a nursing home

HELPFUL HINTS ON GETTING STARTED

Table 2.1 projects the needs of a family support group and provides suggestions for creating an effective group setting.

Because the family support group is an ongoing program, there are many factors to consider to keep the group active from one meeting to the next. Consider the following question very carefully:

- Q: Is it possible that a family support group could fail in the first year?
- A: Yes, but the possibility of failure is greatly diminished when you plan for success.

Take out a pen or marker and underline or highlight the following sentence:

If I plan ahead, the family support group has a better chance of success.

TABLE 2.1. Characteristics of Family Support Group Meetings

Considerations	Suggestions	Anticipated Outcome
physical setting	small library or conference room	cozy, warm, and welcoming
seating arrangements	table with chairs	less intimidating than chairs in a circle
refreshments	sandwiches and beverages	"breaking bread together"
who is invited	families of new admissions in the past year	10 to 15 percent response
method of invitation	assign a family member to send invitations	families connecting = family solidarity
frequency	meet one hour twice a month	more or less often = poor attendance
time/day of week	3 p.m. 1st Tue of month/ 6 p.m. 3rd Tue of month	different time slots = different people
season	year round and reschedule at holidays	loss of momentum = high drop-out rate
facilitator	family co-facilitates w/staff	promotes family ownership/ solidarity

SIX WAYS TO PLAN FOR SUCCESS

Listed below are six ways to plan for a successful family support group. It is essential to be organized from the beginning and to have a plan, to know what is needed to get the group started and how to keep it going. These are six critical elements to consider even before starting a family support group:

- Choosing facilitators
- Building family solidarity
- Marketing the support group
- Preparing an agenda
- Creating a supportive atmosphere
- Communicating outside of support group meetings

Choosing Facilitators

Know the answers to these questions about leadership before you choose facilitators:

- What kind of leadership will allow the greatest flexibility in facilitating the group: laissez-faire, formal versus informal, or authoritative?
- Would the group continue meeting if the staff facilitator became unavailable?
- Are additional staff members available if needed?
- Am I able to attract and draw upon the leadership skills of a family member to help facilitate the group?

The group's ability to stand on its own without the constant support of staff will be a determining factor in the group's rate of success. The staff facilitator must not be viewed as the group's backbone or most important resource. Before the group organizes, plan to solicit at least one family member to be the co-facilitator of the support group. The staff facilitator and co-facilitator should meet regularly to discuss previous group meetings and to make plans for the next scheduled meeting. Part of these plans should include ways to strengthen the co-facilitator's role. Underline or highlight the following sentence:

It may be poor timing to start a support group before attracting a family member to co-facilitate the group.

Building Family Solidarity

Know the answers to these questions about family solidarity before you start the group:

- What kind of feelings do I hope families will have toward one another at the end of each family support group meeting?
- How will I know when family members in the group have bonded?
- How will they act toward each other? What will they say to each other?

- Why is it important for family members to have a sense of community in the nursing home?
- What can I do, as a group facilitator, to promote family solidarity?

One of the main purposes for holding family support groups is to build family solidarity. The support group provides an opportunity for families to connect and bond. In doing so, family members realize they are not alone in the problems or feelings of dealing with a loved one in a nursing home. It is important for the staff facilitator and co-facilitator to recognize the powerful role they play in either building or breaking family solidarity. The facilitators' ability to help members of the group develop a sense of connectedness is another determining factor in the group's rate of success.

One way of helping to build family solidarity is to have the co-facilitator suggest that the support group adopt a name to reflect the group's vision. Some possibilities for names could be: "Helping Hands"; "New Beginnings for Families"; or "Friends of Families." A name other than "Family Support Group" not only makes it easier for families to relate to each other, but is also more descriptive, giving the group character and meaning.

Another way to build family solidarity is to use a vocabulary that will promote the group's image of you as a staff facilitator and not the group's leader. Figure 2.1 provides examples of expressions used by a staff member who is trying to lead the group versus facilitate the group.

FIGURE 2.1. Promoting the Image of Staff Facilitator

Words of a Staff Leader	Words of a Staff Facilitator
I think you should	*What does the **group** think?*
***The** resident, or **our** residents*	***Your** resident*
*In **my** experience*	*What has been **your** experience?*
*The answer to your question **is***	***Who** can help with that question?*
*Your feelings are **normal***	*Has anyone **else** felt this way?*

The words or phrases the staff facilitator and co-facilitator use during support group meetings should cultivate a sense of family togetherness. Thus, the facilitator has the neverending task of using words or phrases that do not sound authoritative. The only true authority on placing a loved one in a nursing home is the person who has successfully done it—not the staff member who has observed it. In a family support group setting, it is more important for families to bond with each other than to bond with staff members. The importance of staff bonding with families and forums that can promote this—are covered in other chapters in this book.

To help facilitators understand how to use a vocabulary that will help family members bond, read the following conversation that occurred at a support group meeting. Use the chart in Figure 2.1 to help pinpoint three words or phrases the facilitator used that failed to express the importance of family solidarity:

Family Member: I'm very upset because my mother doesn't get outside.

Facilitator: I know what you mean. It was so beautiful outside today. Let me talk to the activities department tomorrow about getting the residents outside more often.

The words or phrases in **bold** are the words you should have circled:

I (It isn't important what the facilitator thinks) know what you mean. It was so beautiful outside today.
Let me (Again, the facilitator is owning too much responsibility) talk to the activities department about getting **the residents** (fails to individualize) outside more often.

A more appropriate response might have sounded like this:

Family Member: I'm very upset because my mother doesn't get outside.

Facilitator: It was beautiful outside today, **wasn't it?** (Invites response from the group.) Does **anyone else** wish their resident could be outside more often? (Find out if the problem is an individual issue or broad-based.) **Does anyone** have any ideas about how to solve this problem? (Promotes families to work together on a solution.)

Try again. In the following example, circle at least three words or phrases the facilitator used that failed to express the importance of family solidarity:

Family Member: Every time I visit my mother, she asks me to take her home.

Facilitator: That happens a lot to families. I believe it's just her way of letting you know she's not quite comfortable yet. How does it make you feel when she says that to you? Do you think she understands why you can't take her home?

The words or phrases in **bold** are the words you should have circled:

That **happens a lot** to families. (Fails to individualize.) **I believe it's just her way of letting you know she's not quite comfortable yet.** (The facilitator is acting as the authority.) How does it make **you** (fails to include the group) feel when she says that to you? Do **you** (again, fails to get the group involved in this discussion) think she understands why you can't take her home?

A more appropriate response might have sounded like this:

Has **anyone else** had their resident ask them to take them home? (Find out if the problem is an individual issue or broad-based.) If **the group** had to use one word to describe how it makes you feel when you hear, "take me home," what would that word be? (Talking about feelings as a group is less intimidating than as an individual.) What do **some of you** do when this happens? (Encourages families to share solution-oriented ideas) Does **anyone** have an idea why this happens? (Invites dialogue between family members and keeps the group from looking at the facilitator as the authority.)

Underline or highlight the following sentence:

The support group will have a better chance of success if I plan ahead and develop a vocabulary that will build, not break family solidarity.

The value of planning for a successful family support group cannot be overemphasized. In addition to soliciting family members to co-facilitate and using a vocabulary that builds family solidarity, another critical element to consider before starting the group is a marketing plan.

Marketing the Support Group

Know the answers to these questions about the purpose of a family support group and how to convey this purpose to others:

- What is the nature of the group from a personal standpoint? Why do I want to have a support group at my facility? What personal needs will be fulfilled?
- What professional needs am I fulfilling by offering a family support group?
- In what way will the nursing home benefit by offering a family support group?
- If I were going to attend this support group as a family member, what would need to happen in order for me to feel

comfortable? Would I feel comfortable discussing my feelings?
- What topics would be important to discuss?

Take the time now to reflect upon the above questions and to write your responses on a separate sheet of paper.

The ongoing success of the support group hinges upon your ability to effectively communicate with people about the group. After you have thought about the aforementioned questions, the next step is to discuss these questions with nursing home personnel.

Before your next interdisciplinary care planning meeting, ask the team to set aside ten minutes so that you can discuss your plans to begin a family support group. You should avoid the temptation to provide the staff with written materials about the support group rather than meeting with them. A face-to-face meeting will be much more effective.

When you meet with the team, ask them to answer the following questions:

- How will the residents benefit from a family support group?
- If you were going to attend this support group as a family member, what would need to happen in order for you to feel comfortable? Would you feel comfortable discussing your feelings?
- What topics would be important to discuss?
- How will your department benefit from offering a family support group?

The reason for asking these questions is twofold. First, you want to hear the team's ideas. Each discipline will have a unique perspective on how the nursing home will benefit from a family support group. The opinions expressed will be valuable to you. One idea suggested by a team member may be to use the family support group as a place for family members to air their concerns in a constructive manner. There are times when staff members feel confronted by angry or upset families. If the support group is viewed as a place for families to express these feelings, this may provide relief to a few team members by providing a forum for discussion of family members' concerns.

The second reason for talking to the team about your plans to start a family support group is to educate them. You want the team to realize that the nursing home benefits from having a family support group because the residents will benefit. The more the family is involved in the nursing home, the better the residents' quality of life. It not only raises the residents' spirits to know their families are involved in the different activities of the nursing home, but it also improves the residents' quality of care when the families are more visible. By asking the interdisciplinary team the aforementioned questions, you will demonstrate to the team how important the group is to the nursing home and the residents.

There might be times when you will ask different team members for assistance, and the more they understand the reasons for the support group, the more willing they will be to help. In fact, you may not even have to ask for help, they may volunteer assistance, which is even better. Also, the more team members know about the group, the more likely they will encourage family members to attend.

In addition to asking the interdisciplinary team the aforementioned questions, ask the same questions at a department head meeting. It is important to educate the department heads about the family support group so that they can assist you in marketing the group. Another group of employees for you to consider meeting with is the housekeeping staff. You might not discuss all of the above questions with them, but at least take the time to tell them about the support group. These employees have daily interactions with residents and their families. They see and hear things that other staff members do not. If there is a family member in need of attending the support group, the housekeepers may know about it. Underline or highlight the following sentence:

The support group will have a better chance of success if I talk to other staff members about the purpose of the support group.

Once you have spoken with the staff about the support group, the next step is to inform family members about the group. To start a family support group, send formal invitations to family members of residents who were admitted to the nursing home during the past year. Thereafter, at the time of each new admission, written information should be given to family members concerning the family support group. A brief paragraph explaining the purpose of the group and when it meets is all that is needed at this time. Families are often inundated with paperwork at the time of admission, and this is not the ideal time to call their attention to the group. It will be more effective to share information about the support group at a later time.

At the time of admission, mention to the family members that they may be receiving an invitation to attend a support group during the next month. Explain that family involvement is especially critical during the resident's first month of admission. To help facilitate the resident's adjustment, the nursing home recommends that family attend at least one support group meeting. If a family member has not attended the group in the first one or two months of admission, ask the support group to send that family member a formal invitation to attend. Sometimes receiving an invitation from a fellow family member may be more meaningful than receiving an invitation from a staff member. See the Appendix for a sample invitation.

It is of significance to note that a resident's spouse may instinctively include the resident as part of the invitation to attend the support group. If you do not clearly state that the support group is not for the residents themselves, you may find yourself in an awkward position when a spouse shows up at one of the meetings with his or her resident.

Once the support group has been explained to family members and invitations have been sent out, it is important to continuously remind families and staff when the meetings are to be held. Posters should be placed in the nursing home lobby one week before each support group meeting. Local radio stations may also be willing to announce the date and time of each group meeting. In smaller communities, the local newspaper may be interested in featuring a story about the support group.

Marketing strategies will contribute significantly to the initial success of the support group. Even though you may feel uncertain about your first try at a support group, do not hesitate to market the group. Marketing is one of the most important actions you will take as you plan for the support group.

A fourth critical element to consider before the family support group begins is a list of topics to be discussed at the group meetings. In order to successfully get group members to disclose their concerns, an agenda should be prepared. Facilitators should come to meetings prepared to present a topic to discuss.

Preparing an Agenda

Know the answers to these questions about preparing an agenda before you start the group.

- As a facilitator, if I must choose, will the group focus on a preestablished agenda or will each meeting be informal with no particular topic planned.
- If there is an agenda, should the group be expected to follow the agenda or can group members just talk about whatever is on their minds?
- Who should plan the agenda or topics for discussion?

One of the main purposes for holding a family support group is to provide a comforting atmosphere in which families can progress through the different stages of adjustment. Subsequently, families will learn how to manage the problems of and/or feelings toward having a loved one in a nursing home. It is important for the facilitators to know how to use an agenda to create such an atmosphere. In order to plan an agenda, the facilitator should understand the various stages of adjustment to nursing home placement. See Table 2.2 for a description of the different stages of adjustment and related topics for discussion.

Not every family member will go through each stage in the order presented in Table 2.2. However, the staff facilitator should be aware of what stage each family member is in and whether he or she is "stuck" in one particular stage or has moved through stages rather quickly. For example, a family member whose resident was admitted in the past two weeks would not be at a stage of acceptance without having recognized and dealt with some of the losses that have occurred. If you note such a family member attending the support group, a topic for discussion might be, "How my daily routine changed when (mother) was admitted to the nursing home." This question may help the family member realize how much worry and responsibility he or she had prior to placement. If you notice that a family member is in a pattern of self-criticism or feels guilty for not taking care of his or her loved one at home, you might plan a topic, such as, "What is the definition of guilt?" People often hide behind words such as guilt without dealing with their true feelings.

Planning an agenda should take into consideration the factors that are influencing each family member's ability to move through the different stages of adjustment. However, if the support group is open to new members, then certain formalities must precede a planned agenda. If the support group is not closed to new members, certain topics need to be discussed at the beginning of each meeting to accommodate newcomers.

TABLE 2.2. Stages of Adjustment and Related Topics for Discussion

Stage I	Denial	• Denying the loss that occurs after placing a loved one in a nursing home • Failing to notice the changes in the family after placing a loved one • Denying the right to be free from guilt and self-criticism
	Topics to Discuss	• "How has the family's daily routine changed since placement?" • "What role does the family have in the nursing home?" • "Were the circumstances that led to placement avoidable?"
Stage II	Guilt and Anger	• Anger at other family members for not helping with the placement process • Anger at staff for seemingly not accommodating the resident's needs • Anger at the resident for not accepting placement and blaming family
	Topics to Discuss	• "What is the definition of guilt?" • "How to tell someone you're angry." • "How to know when you've done your best." • "What is another word for anger?"
Stage III	Sadness and Grief	• Acknowledging a separation and loss • Recognizing and working through feelings such as guilt and self-criticism • Realizing the negative effects of placement
	Topics to Discuss	• "How have other family members gotten through the grief?" • "What is another word for sadness?" • "How can the losses associated with placement be replaced?"
Stage IV	Acceptance	• Turning to the future and learning what can and cannot be changed • Recognizing placement was the best choice, given the circumstances
	Topics to Discuss	• "What are the positive and negative effects of nursing home placement?" • "When do you know the nursing home is doing its best?" • "What words of advice can you give to other families adjusting to placement?"

The first time a family member comes to the support group, he or she should be introduced, and a description of the circumstances that led to nursing home placement for his or her loved one should be given. If there is more than one new family member at a meeting, this task may take up most of the group's time. This is acceptable on occasion; however, enough time should remain to discuss the planned topic. As the newcomer describes the circumstances that led to placement, the facilitators should be assessing in which stage of adjustment the newcomer is. If introducing new members is taking up most of the group's time, you may want to suggest that the group meet for more than one hour.

Another possibility is to close the group to new members and start an additional group to accommodate them. Because the support group will become less intimate as the group grows larger, it is advisable to start an additional group for newcomers if there are more than ten members regularly attending the original group. If there are a number of families from one particular unit of the nursing home who are interested in attending a support group, it is beneficial to keep them in the same group. For example, families who have residents on a special care unit for treatment of dementia will have more in common with each other than with families who have residents with no cognitive impairment.

Before you start a support group, become familiar with the different stages of adjustment. On an ongoing basis, evaluate what stage each group member is working on. Underline or highlight the following sentence:

> *An agenda can be used to help family members move through the different stages of adjustment.*

Creating a supportive atmosphere takes more time and planning than preparing topics for discussion. The facilitators must also think about how to keep the group comfortable and purposeful and how to keep group members thinking constructive, positive thoughts. The fifth critical element to consider as you plan to start a support group is how to create a supportive atmosphere.

Creating a Supportive Atmosphere

Before starting a support group, know the answers to these questions about creating a supportive atmosphere in which family members can discuss their concerns:

- What does a supportive atmosphere feel like? What does it look like? What does it sound like?
- Should families be expected to give as well as receive support? What should be done if one family member seems always to be on the receiving end?
- How deeply should feelings be explored, and should there be therapeutic exercises to get families in touch with feelings they don't even know they have?
- What can be done when the group is airing their concerns but there doesn't seem to be any resolution, when the focus of the group's discussion becomes problem oriented?

Take the time now to reflect on the above questions. If you have thought through these questions first, it will help in achieving your vision of what the support group should be. Share these questions with the co-facilitator before starting the family support group. It is important for the facilitators to agree on ways to create a supportive atmosphere.

Both facilitators must agree that the support group is not group therapy. The family support group is not the appropriate forum to analyze family dynamics and/or seek to change individual personalities. Although the support group will discuss topics that are therapeutic, family members are not seeking therapy by attending a support group. The support group is a place for family members to exchange information and share common experiences while giving mutual support.

Therapeutic exercises to bring out feelings may serve only one or two members of the group and may make others feel uncomfortable. When the support group meets, avoid asking probing questions that are meant to examine and expose deep emotional turmoil. For example, avoid questions such as, "It must be really hard for you to be looking after your mother now, when she neglected you all those years." Long-standing emotional problems or severe family problems are best dealt with in a more structured atmosphere, such as individual counseling or group therapy.

Through the natural course of the group process, families may indeed "get in touch with their feelings." "Getting in touch with feelings" is not why families will say they are coming to the group, and facilitators should agree it is not a primary purpose. Underline or highlight the following sentence:

> *Families will keep coming to the group if they feel comfortable.*

Facilitators must also recognize the importance of creating an environment that promotes mutual assistance. Your plan should be to create a friendly, supportive environment in which people feel they are connected to others in the "same boat." You will have successfully promoted mutual assistance if family members express gratitude for having a place to talk about their concerns and feelings. The group may be the only place for families to come and be with other people who understand the impact of placing a loved one in a nursing home. Group members often feel that their friends or other members of the family are tired of hearing about it or would not understand to begin with. If members view the group's purpose as an opportunity to come together for mutual assistance, then there will be a higher level of commitment and attendance. Take out a pen or marker and highlight the following sentence:

Members of the group will feel purposeful if there is mutual assistance.

To create a supportive environment the facilitators must have a plan to avoid the "gripevine." Concerns being raised will grow into a "gripevine" if the group fails to provide a supportive atmosphere. It is important to acknowledge a concern that is brought to the group, but the focus should be on the solution, not the problem. Describing the problem in great detail and trying to figure out the cause of the problem will leave little time to talk about the solution. Focusing on the problem and not the solution will cause the group to become frustrated and discontent. If the "gripevine" continues to grow over several meetings, family members may begin to lose interest. The attendance at the support group meetings will dwindle, if not abruptly end. If families leave the group feeling dissatisfied and feeling that they have no constructive place to voice their concerns, then they may not only give up on the group, but they may also feel the need to take their concerns elsewhere, such as to a local newspaper or an advocacy agency. Underline or highlight the following sentence:

The difference between an unsupportive atmosphere and a supportive atmosphere is that the former focuses on the problem while the latter focuses on the solution.

A plan to avoid the "gripevine" should include recognizing the value of family members sharing similar experiences. Once a concern has been raised, the facilitator should determine if it is an individual concern or a broad-based concern: "Has anyone else experienced this problem?" Before discussion, it is important to know how many group members are afflicted with the problem. Knowing ahead of time how many members have a particular problem will also tell you how much time to spend on the issue. If it is an individual problem, less time will be spent in discussion than if it is broad based.

Because people are sometimes more convinced by suggestions made by others than suggestions they devise on their own, always ask the group for suggestions on how to deal with an individual concern or a broad-based problem. The group may not offer a novel idea, but may only reaffirm for members what they already know.

Often, problems get adequately addressed when other members share their experiences of how they overcame similar circumstances. This approach works well because the support group is comprised of individuals who are at different stages of the adjustment process. The co-facilitator or other family members who have had a loved one in the nursing home for several months will want to be helpful to the newer members of the group. They will have "cleared some hurdles" and will want to share how they did it.

For example, if a new family member mentions to the group that he or she is feeling overwhelmed and also indicates that he or she is visiting twice a day, other family members will have ideas, based on experience, about reducing the amount of time being spent at the facility. Remember, family members will tell you one of the reasons they keep coming to the group is because they feel needed or purposeful. One of the ways they feel purposeful is by helping fellow group members. Underline or highlight the following sentence:

Members of the group will feel purposeful if there are opportunities to give.

As was just discussed, one way of avoiding the "gripevine" and keeping the group solution-oriented is to have members who are at different stages of adjustment share their experiences and how they overcame similar problems. This method works well, but there are times when discussions will stray and become less constructive and more problem-oriented. At such times a "tool-box" may be required to get the group back on track. A "toolbox" is similar to a carpenter's toolbox, in which tools can be found to make, build, or repair something that is not working. Facilitators need to be sensitive to the warning signs that indicate when a group is disintegrating. Poor attendance, monotonous, dreary discussions, and poor eye contact are all warning signs that should alert the facilitators to reach into the toolbox to help refocus the discussion.

Preparing a Toolbox

There should be at least three or four ideas in the toolbox to use when the group is in need of something new and different. These tools will guide the group toward more constructive, solution-oriented discussion. Both facilitators should work together to prepare the toolbox before beginning a family support group. Depending on your style and the group's characteristics, here are some ideas to consider for the toolbox.

Tool #1. The Gift of Wishes

This technique gives members an opportunity to exercise their imagination and bestow goodwill to other group members. Giving the "Gift of Wishes" (see Figure 2.2) not only brightens up the group discussion, but validates concerns. For example, family members who express fear about a hereditary disease will be wished "good health" by other group members. A resident's spouse who is afraid to go on a vacation will be wished "peace of

FIGURE 2.2. The Gift of Wishes

FOR YOUR RESIDENT I WISH...

FOR YOU I WISH...

mind." A family member who is not accustomed to having free time will be wished "a new and exciting hobby." Wishes can also be given to the family member's resident.

The "Gift of Wishes" is especially good to take out of the toolbox when a family member is having a difficult time and the group is at a loss for words. Do not single out the family member who is having a difficult time by having the group give the "Gift of Wishes" only to that individual. Each member should receive and give a wish. You can accomplish this by having each member give "The Gift of Wishes" to the person on his or her left. Figure 2.2 should be copied ahead of time onto colored paper and placed in the toolbox for future use.

Tool #2. Role Modeling

This technique is effective because the group focuses on a problem by looking at it from someone else's point of view. Place in your toolbox names of people who are likely to be well-known by those attending the group. Perhaps these people are known figures of the community, such as a doctor, mayor, police chief, clergy, farmer, or teacher. These people may also include television personalities, national politicians, professional artists, or athletes and coaches.

When you have determined that the group has strayed and is in need of a positive influence, pull a person's name out of the toolbox. The name you use should be someone the group can relate to and have positive feelings about. Write this person's name on a chalkboard or easel and draw three large boxes above the name. Ask the group to fill each box with a word or phrase that best describes this person's beliefs about how to overcome problems in life. The following questions might generate some ideas: Does this person believe that things happen by chance or things happen by taking action? In this person's opinion, what is probably the best way to approach problems: head-on or through the back door? How would this person complete this sentence, "Life is like . . ."?

Once you have filled the three boxes, at the bottom of the diagram write the problem the group was having trouble constructively discussing. For example, let's say a family member who is visiting the nursing home, sometimes twice a day, was talking about feeling overwhelmed with responsibility. She feels responsible for placing a loved one in the nursing home and if anything goes wrong she will feel at fault. This family member's husband wants to take a vacation for the first time in years, but she is afraid to leave things in the hands of the nursing home. Ask the group to imagine how the person named in the diagram would approach this problem. Look at the boxes and apply the problem to the statements in boxes. Figure 2.3 is an example of this technique.

Sometimes the group may still have trouble focusing on the

FIGURE 2.3. Diagrams to Use to Approach the Feeling of Being Overwhelmed with Responsibility

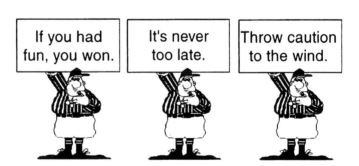

WHAT WOULD THE WINNINGEST COACH IN FOOTBALL HISTORY SAY ABOUT FEELING OVERWHELMED WITH RESPONSIBILITY?

solution rather than the problem. Because of all your planning, it is unlikely that the group will reach such a level of frustration but if it does, you must reach into your toolbox and try something different.

Tool #3. *Redefining Words That Describe Feelings*

During group meetings, a problem will often be expressed by using words that describe a feeling. One of the greatest tools to use to help the group communicate and understand each other is to define a word or phrase. The phrase "overwhelmed with responsibility" may not mean the same thing to everyone in the group. In many cases, definitions represent different feelings for different members. A problem feels different when someone says "anger means resentment" or "guilt means shame" because the individual is clarifying his or her feelings.

One way to help the group stay constructive and solution oriented is to determine what a specific word or phrase means to the group. This can be done by asking the group to use alternative words to define a feeling. Facilitators should never assume how the group defines a word. Place in your toolbox a list of words describing various emotions. Next to these words write down alternatives. Use this list when the support group has difficulty thinking of alternatives. For example:

Feeling	Alternative definitions	
anger	resentment	annoyed upset
guilt	ashamed	broken promises
overwhelmed	exhausted	defeated

If a family member tells the group he is feeling overwhelmed with responsibility ask, "What does overwhelmed mean?" If the group is unable to brainstorm and redefine "overwhelmed," consult your list.

When the group defines a feeling, the solution to the problem becomes more clear. For example, if a group member says, "overwhelmed means feeling tired," then ask, "What is the answer to feeling tired?" It is easier to think of a solution to being tired than it is to think of a solution to being overwhelmed.

Another word you will redefine often is "complain." When a family member says, "I hate to complain but . . ." plan to respond with, "It's not a complaint; it's a concern." Using a less coarse word validates the family member's feelings, lessens the intensity of the problem, and encourages members to continue voicing their concerns.

Tool #4. Changing the Focus

Another item to place in the toolbox is a list of techniques to change the focus of a discussion. If the group has become problem oriented, then do something that takes the focus away from the problem. This does not necessarily mean changing the subject, but rather changing the image of the problem. Sometimes in order to change the focus you must do something unexpected. While doing something unexpected, try to capitalize on the group's sense of humor. Scientific studies have demonstrated that laughter is cathartic and causes a chemical reaction that generates positive thoughts and feelings.

For example, as a facilitator you notice that the support group has been trying to help a family member. This family member is overcome with guilt feelings for having broken a promise to keep a loved one out of a nursing home. Tell the group that the problem they are discussing reminds you of an *I Love Lucy* episode. Suddenly, group members are thinking of a funny redheaded lady. In fact, pull out a picture of Lucy from the toolbox.

Ask the group if they see how Lucy's problems might be similar to the problem being discussed by the support group. Lucy was known for getting herself into predicaments by making promises she could not possibly keep. Ask the group if they can recall any such episodes. If the group cannot recall an episode, have a few written examples in your toolbox ready to use. After describing an *I Love Lucy* episode, ask the group if they agree that Lucy tended to make promises she couldn't keep? Why did she do that? What does the family member who made a promise to never place a loved one in a nursing home have in common with Lucy? The purpose of relating the group's discussion to an *I Love Lucy* episode is to change the image of the problem by tapping into the group's sense of humor.

If the support group lacks a sense of humor, then the facilitator should have a more serious approach available in the toolbox. A more serious way to change the image of a problem is to have the group intellectualize the problem as an opportunity to learn. This is based on the philosophy that there is no such thing as a problem, only opportunities to learn. However, this tool only works if the problem is indeed a problem. For example, a family member who visits the nursing home twice a day may not look upon this frequency of visiting as a problem. Perhaps it is only a problem for nursing staff or for a spouse at home who is feeling neglected. Always ask first, "Whose problem is it?"

If a family member has established that visiting his or her resident twice a day is a problem, one technique of keeping the focus solution-oriented would be to have the group apply the phrase, "Lessons in life often appear as problems." Reach into your toolbox and bring out an index card on which the following phrase is written: "Lessons in life often appear as problems."

For example, a family member is feeling guilty for placing a loved one in the nursing home because a promise was made to always care for the loved one at home. Ask a member to read the card to the group, "Lessons in life often appear as problems." What is the lesson to learn about making promises? Underline or highlight the following sentence:

The support group will have a better chance of success if there are tools readily available to help keep the group's focus constructive, solution oriented, and based on mutual assistance.

Creating a supportive atmosphere requires the facilitators to consider ways to keep the group comfortable, *purposeful*, and effective. The sixth critical element to consider as you plan to start a support group is how to keep the lines of communication open between support group meetings.

Communicating Outside of Support Group Meetings

Before starting a support group, know the answers to these questions about communicating with family members outside of group meetings:

- Should group members be discouraged from discussing issues with each other outside of the meetings?
- Should a group member be approached by a facilitator to privately discuss an issue that was brought up during a meeting?

One of the purposes of holding a family support group is to help build family solidarity. Families should not have to wait for a meeting to discuss their concerns or to get questions answered. The lines of communication should be kept open between meetings. One way of doing this is to have a mailbox at the facility for the co-facilitator, who is also a family member. This way family members can communicate with each other between meetings, and they do not have to wait for a meeting to reach out to one another.

If a family member appears upset or unsettled at the end of a group meeting, the facilitators should offer to meet privately with this family member. In some cases you may even want to try to set up a meeting with an individual family member and other staff members if an unresolved problem seems to involve other disciplines and the resident's provision of care. Underline or highlight the following sentence:

> *The ability of the family member to successfully deal with the problems of and feelings toward having a loved one in a nursing home is directly related to keeping lines of communication open during and between family support group meetings.*

This chapter covered the critical elements needed to create a supportive atmosphere in which family members can talk openly about their concerns and feelings about having a loved one in a nursing home. In starting a family support group, the value of planning for success cannot be overemphasized. The plan may include, but is not limited to, the following elements: choosing a family member to co-facilitate; building family solidarity; marketing and educating others about the group; preparing an agenda; creating a supportive atmosphere that is based on mutual assistance and focused on solutions; and keeping the lines of communication open. The support group provides family members the opportunity to react to a problem or feeling and then focus on a solution.

The next chapter on Family Councils encompasses a different approach to problem solving. The Family Council plays a proactive role in helping to deter or avoid ordinary problems commonly faced in the nursing home.

Chapter 3

Family Councils

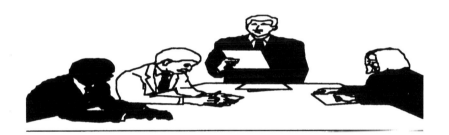

PURPOSE OF THE FAMILY COUNCIL

- To encourage shared decision-making in the operations of the nursing home
- To positively affect the job satisfaction of nursing home employees
- To improve the residents' quality of life
- To expand the role and responsibilities of families in the nursing home

WHAT CAN BE GAINED BY SPONSORING A FAMILY COUNCIL

The concept behind sponsoring a Family Council is for the nursing home to provide families with the opportunity to play a proactive role in the operation of the nursing home. Thus, families can positively affect the residents' life and the services provided. Through the Family Council, the nursing home gains a unique spirit, one that reflects a nature of shared decision-making. Having a Family Council keeps the lines of communication open between staff members and families. When families have a voice in operational decisions and feel their suggestions are seriously considered, then families will be less likely to be dissatisfied or take their concerns elsewhere. In essence, by sponsoring a Family Council, the nursing home incites a partnership between the staff and family in providing above-average service for the residents.

HOW A FAMILY COUNCIL IS FORMED

Staff from different disciplines should select three to five family members to meet and discuss forming a Family Council. These family members are designated as officers and, with the assistance of a staff liaison, are responsible for organizing a Family Council. The total family population is invited to Family Council meetings with the officers presiding over each meeting. Officers will perform the duties and functions of the traditional Chair, Co-Chair, Secretary, and Treasurer. Once the Council becomes well-established, a decision can be made concerning the duration of each officer's term. The importance of having officers cannot be overemphasized. If a team of family members cannot be found to serve as leaders, it may not be worthwhile to start a Family Council.

HELPFUL HINTS ON GETTING STARTED

Table 3.1 projects the needs of a Family Council and provides suggestions on creating an atmosphere that is formal and business-oriented. One of the most common mistakes made in meeting the needs of a Family Council is permitting a lack of formal-

TABLE 3.1. Characteristics of Family Council Meetings

Considerations	Suggestions	Anticipated Outcome
physical setting	small library or conference room	good ventilation and space
seating arrangements	tables with chairs	induces formality
refreshments	beverages only	more business-like
# invited to council	interested families	15-33 percent response
method of invitation	mailings/posters	encourages participation of all families
frequency/duration of meeting	1.5 hours every month	allows time for old and new business
time/day of week	late afternoon or early evening	council members choose
season	year-round and reschedule at holidays	consistent attendance/ commitment
speakers	administration and other staff when invited	induces formality/ accountability

ity. A formal atmosphere will assure follow-through. Skipping meetings over the summer or not rescheduling after a holiday is not advisable. If council meetings are held too far apart, then family members will lose interest. If meetings are not held in a timely manner, family members will not realize the cause and effect of the Council's efforts. After the Council has met two or three times, a decision should be made on how often to hold general meetings. If general meetings are held quarterly, the officers still need to meet monthly.

WHAT THE FAMILY COUNCIL WILL DO

The Family Council will stimulate change in the nursing home. The Council will examine current policies and procedures and recommend changes toward achieving the nursing home's mission statement. Mission statements almost always focus on being dedicated to delivering efficient, dependable, and timely service. The Family Council will make observations of the care and services being provided in the nursing home and will provide feedback to the nursing home staff about their observations. Underline or highlight the following sentence:

> *The nursing home that welcomes change will seek the vision of a Family Council.*

The nursing home will consult the Family Council prior to making operational changes. For example, if a decision was made to close the dining room whenever staffing is low and to serve meals in the residents' rooms, the nursing home would consult the Council before implementing the new policy. The Council's permission is not required before the nursing home institutes new policies and procedures; however, the Council's response to proposed changes must be seriously considered by the administration. Underline or highlight the following sentence:

The nursing home that wishes to inspire a higher level of accountability will seek the voice of a Family Council.

WHAT YOU NEED TO BEGIN

A Staff Liaison

Presumably, the reader of this book will serve as the staff liaison. The purpose of the liaison is to help build an alliance between the Family Council and the administration and staff of the nursing home. The liaison will initially attend the first two meetings to help with organizational procedures. This will include ensuring the election of officers, explaining the roles and responsibilities of each officer, and providing information about the overall purpose of the Family Council. In selecting officers, it is preferable to have each wing or unit of the nursing home represented. Family members who attend council meetings should realize their efforts will be directed not only toward their resident, but toward the good of all the residents in the nursing home.

The staff liaison may need to help the Family Council realize its role as a change agent and to understand that Council meetings should focus on proactive issues. Meetings will center on improving the residents' quality of life and methods of raising or maintaining staff morale. Families may air their concerns at council meetings, but these concerns need to be followed up with suggestions, and in some cases, offers to help. The staff liaison will find it helpful to review Chapter 2 of this book, particularly the section on avoiding the "gripevine."

After the second or third meeting, the Council should consider the necessity of having the liaison stay throughout each meeting. Councils that are without strong family leaders would obviously benefit from having the staff liaison at each meeting; however, such a council should continuously work toward having some time at each meeting when there is no staff member present. If there are family members willing and able to lead the council meetings, then the liaison need only be present for a small portion of each meeting. Ideally, the liaison should offer support and availability at the beginning and/or end of each meeting. At the very least, the liaison should be in the building whenever the Council is holding a meeting. If the Council has any questions or concerns, the liaison should be readily accessible.

A Resource Team

The Family Council will need a team of resourceful people who can be available when needed. These individuals will form a committee called the Resource Team, and the Council can utilize the expertise of this team. The Resource Team will be comprised of individuals who hold positions at the nursing home and have the following useful qualities: managerial and economic power (administration); advocacy abilities (residents, social workers); direct-care experience (nursing staff); connections with the community (board members or trustees); and theoretical and philosophical perspectives on how to meet the needs of nursing home residents (clergy, physicians). It is the job of the staff liaison to assemble a group of individuals willing to serve on the Resource Team. After such a team has been established, the Resource Team should inform the Family Council of its availability. The following letter is an example of how the Resource Team may do this:

Dear Family Council Members:

On behalf of the Resource Team, we welcome you to the Family Council. We are a team of individuals who, like yourself, are committed to providing services consistent with the residents' everchanging needs. We believe that through combined efforts, the Family Council and the

Resource Team cultivate compassion, expertise, and excellence–all necessary ingredients in providing the residents with a higher quality of care. We invite you to call on us whenever you need assistance, and we will do whatever we can to accommodate you. The Resource Team is specifically designed to respond to your needs with expedience, effectiveness, and even imagination. We are here as your ally and have pledged to do our best to support you. Please do not hesitate to contact us if you would like the Resource Team or any member of the team to attend one of your Family Council meetings or to assist you in any other way.

Sincerely yours,

Administrator / Staff Liaison / Resident Council Member / Nursing Administration / Quality Assurance Committee Member / Employee of the Year / Board Member or Trustee / Clergy / Certified Nurse's Aide / Physician / Coordinator of Volunteer Services

The liaison should encourage the Family Council to ask for the Resource Team's input as frequently as possible. Ideas for when and how to involve the Resource Team are discussed later in this chapter, but the Council should not be limited to these suggestions.

A Funding Plan

The Family Council will need money to purchase supplies, finance new projects, and support additional endeavors. Uses for money will be thoroughly explained later in this chapter. The Council will need to know what portion of its financial needs can be met by the nursing home. It is likely that the nursing home will not be able to meet all the financial requirements of the Council; however, the nursing home should make a contribution, especially when the Council is in the beginning stages. The size of the contribution is not as important as the gesture. Any contribution demonstrates a commitment by the nursing home to support and sanction the Council's efforts.

With a little creative thinking, most of the Council's financial needs will be met through fund-raisers and donations made by public and private organizations. The key to financial and organizational success is for the Council and the Resource Team to pool their resources and work together. The Council should hold a meeting with the Resource Team to generate ideas for fund-raisers and to identify names of individuals and organizations willing to provide financial or material resources.

A Schedule of Events

Although the Family Council should work toward being self-governing, the staff liaison must provide guidance and direction in the beginning stages. The Council may not know how to proceed once it starts to organize. Therefore, the staff liaison must provide a schedule of events so the Council's activities can remain structured and purposeful. The schedule of events will be provided to the Council with the understanding that it is not unchangeable. In fact, the schedule is *expected* to be altered, according to the Council's needs and wishes. If the Family Council meets quarterly, council members may need to form subcommittees to organize monthly events. A suggested schedule of events is illustrated in Figure 3.1. It is important to note that these are possible activities and the Council should not limit themselves to only these suggestions.

DESCRIPTION OF SCHEDULED EVENTS

Bulletin Boards

Each month the Family Council will be responsible for decorating a bulletin board. The bulletin board can be used to adver-

FIGURE 3.1. Family Council Schedule of Events

January	February	March	April
Bulletin Board	Bulletin Board	Bulletin Board	Bulletin Board
Panel Discussion		Pancake Breakfast	Holiday Social
May	**June**	**July**	**August**
No Bulletin Board	Bulletin Board	Bulletin Board	Bulletin Board
Fund Raiser		Scavenger Hunt	
September	**October**	**November**	**December**
No Bulletin Board	Bulletin Board	Bulletin Board	Bulletin Board
Fund Raiser		Adopt-a-Resident	Holiday Social

tise upcoming events, celebrate holidays, keep track of announcements, display thankful notes to staff, or showcase "People You Should Know." The nursing home should offer to pay for the bulletin board of the Council's choice. The materials used to decorate the bulletin boards will be paid for by the Council. Once in a while the Council should be given a break from decorating the bulletin board and staff (and/or residents) could offer to do it instead.

Fund-Raisers

Fund-raisers such as car washes, bottle recycling, and bake sales, work well for a variety of reasons. Besides raising money, fund-raisers bring residents, families, and staff closer together in a common effort. Fund-raisers also promote a favorable relationship between the nursing home and the community. Other ideas for fund-raisers include the following: a talent show starring families, residents, and staff; a casino night with card games, bingo, and 50/50 raffle tickets; or a sports tournament night with residents and family members challenging staff in games such as balloon volleyball, wheelchair basketball, or shuffleboard.

A Holiday Scavenger Hunt

A scavenger hunt can be organized to help celebrate a holiday such as Independence Day. The idea is to collect certain items relative to the holiday, and then use these items to decorate the nursing home. The Resource Team and Family Council will meet and divide into teams, and a captain is chosen for each. Each team will choose a unit of the nursing home to decorate. The captain will ask the staff and residents of each unit to join the scavenger team. The corridors, the residents' doors, and/or dining/lounge area will be decorated with the items collected by the scavenger hunt team. Each unit will be open for display on the holiday.

Money should not be used to purchase all of the items, but each scavenger hunt team will have some money to use from the Family Council fund. Many of the items could be brought in from people's homes. For example, items such as flags, scarves, food, clothes, trinkets, music, and decorations can usually be found at home. Some of the items can be posters drawn by team members. Each scavenger hunt team will make or collect items related to a theme that represents the holiday. For example, to celebrate Independence Day, teams could decorate one unit with a red, white, and blue theme, while another team uses a theme that includes patriotic music and other sounds. Staff, residents, and families may choose to dress in costumes on the day each unit will be displayed.

The team captains should meet with the Resident Council one month prior to the scavenger hunt. The purpose of meeting with the Resident Council is to encourage resident participation and to find out if they would like the final decorations to be judged. For example, awards could be given for different categories depending on the scavenger hunt theme.

Each year the Family Council will pick a different holiday for the scavenger hunt. It is best to pick holidays that usually have a low profile in nursing homes, such as Halloween, St. Patrick's Day, or Valentine's Day. The more visible families are during holidays, the more home-like the atmosphere will be.

A Pancake Breakfast

Once a year the Family Council should sponsor a staff appreciation day. One way of doing this is for the Family Council to invite the staff to a pancake breakfast. The entire staff will be invited, and staff members should be encouraged to bring a guest. The Council will purchase, prepare, and serve the breakfast at a local church or club if it cannot be done at the nursing home. If any of the Family Council members are musically inclined, and a large group is expected, musical entertainment could also be provided. Council members might also consider making small speeches about how much the staff is appreciated. For those staff members who are unable to attend the breakfast because they are working, the Family Council could bring pastries to each unit/wing of the nursing home.

Adopt-a-Resident

November and December are difficult months for residents who have no visitors. These residents could be identified for the Family Council so that each member can adopt a resident during these difficult months. It is not imperative that the identified residents be cognitively intact—as long as they can respond appropriately to the Council member's visits.

Council members who adopt a resident are given the handout "How To Make Visits Count" to use as a resource. This handout is found in the Appendix. Council members will visit these residents regularly throughout November and December. The residents who are visited should be told from the beginning that the

Family Council has designated November and December as a special time to get acquainted. Council members who are visiting these residents may decide to continue visiting past December, but should be warned against making promises concerning how often they will visit.

At the beginning of January, the adopted residents and council members should come together for a special meeting with a member of the clergy. Council members may not be able to continue visiting these residents throughout the year, so the purpose of the meeting is to help these residents connect with one another. At the beginning of the meeting, the clergyperson tells the residents what they all have in common (i.e., they have all just spent two months getting acquainted with members of the Family Council). Family Council members should then stand, introduce themselves, and thank the residents for spending time with them. Next, residents should be prompted to introduce themselves. Then the nursing home Chaplin or clergyperson should give a short sermon that addresses the following topic: "Today, no matter who I'm with, I will think, 'How can I be of service to others?' " The emphasis should be on how residents can help each other.

After this message all the residents are helped to form a circle. Have the residents hold a piece of ribbon long enough to go around the circle. The ribbon signifies oneness among the residents. Family Council members should stand behind the residents and not hold the ribbon. While the residents hold the ribbon, a song such as "Side-by-Side" could be sung by all. To illustrate the residents' connectedness, council members should pin a piece of the same colored ribbon (but not the ribbon the residents are holding) to each resident's collar or blouse. While the council members do this, the Chaplin will give a benediction. At the conclusion of the Chaplin's blessing, the doors will be opened so that all residents in the facility can join the others for an ice cream social.

Panel Discussions

At least once a year, the Family Council should invite the nursing home administrator and department heads to attend a council meeting for a panel discussion. The purpose is for the Family Council to give staff input concerning their impressions of the nursing home. This input will include praise as well as constructive criticisms of areas that are in need of improvement. If preferred, a list of questions can be developed by the Council and given to the staff ahead of time. Any new or additional questions can be submitted to the panel on index cards.

Council members may want to concentrate on issues that have been mentioned at previous council meetings. General comments could also be shared concerning the overall care and appearance of the nursing home. The following list of questions can be used to generate discussion:

- Does the nursing home seem comfortable and home-like?
- Are there any problems with missing belongings or clothing?
- Is there usually a private place to visit?
- Is the noise level appropriate?
- Are the residents well groomed, clean, shaven, and appropriately dressed?
- Do the residents have enough activity? Are there suggestions for other types of activities?
- Are the residents being encouraged to do enough for themselves?
- Are the residents getting the assistance they need?
- Are residents treated with dignity and respect?
- Are call lights answered in a timely fashion?
- Are the residents in good spirits?
- Do the staff members keep families notified of the residents' condition?
- Do staff members welcome family visits?

• Is there anything else the staff should know about families perceptions of the nursing home?

The panel discussion is facilitated by the Council, but administration plays an important role throughout the meeting. The role of the administrator is to promote open lines of communication between council members and staff. The administrator will thank the Council for the opportunity to attend a council meeting. The administrator should also stress the importance of staff and family working together to provide the residents with a better quality of life.

At the conclusion of the panel discussion, the nursing home's mission statement could be displayed on an overhead. Mission statements usually include a philosophy about being dedicated to delivering efficient, dependable, and timely service. Looking at the mission statement and taking the preceding discussion into consideration, the administrator, panel of department heads and Family Council members could reflect on the nursing home's strengths and weaknesses. If the mission statement is not being achieved, and there are several concerns, it would be beneficial to hold another panel discussion within three to six months. The Resource Team and the Family Council can also make arrangements to work together on solving some of the identified problems. If the mission statement is being achieved, then new goals could be discussed with the Family Council. The Family Council may want to show the nursing home its appreciation by sending a letter to the local advocacy agency describing the good care the residents are receiving at the nursing home. Although complaints are primarily filed, these agencies are also interested in hearing positive reports from families who are involved in nursing homes.

Holiday Socials

Another way to reach out to the total family population is to offer families the opportunity to get together with the residents to celebrate a special event. At least twice a year, the Family Council will sponsor a Holiday Social. Family members who have shown no interest in attending formal family meetings, such as support groups, councils, or educational workshops, might enjoy getting together under more casual, less structured circumstances.

Although staff will provide assistance, it is important that the Family Council host or sponsor Holiday Socials. The Family Council sets an example for other family members regarding involvment in the nursing home as a leader and/or participant. A family member will likely feel a stronger sense of belonging when he or she observes other family members having an effective influence upon the nursing home. The more family members demonstrate their leadership ability to the family population, the more comfortable families will feel about operational decisions and proposed policy changes in the nursing home.

If there is one factor that elevates a nursing home out of the ordinary, it is the level of family involvement at the nursing home. An active Family Council is one way to positively affect the residents' lives and the services provided in the nursing home. Through the Family Council, the nursing home gains a unique spirit, one that reflects a nature of shared decision making and commitment in meeting the needs of the residents.

The next chapter provides you with more detailed information on bringing families together for a Holiday Social.

Chapter 4

Holiday Socials

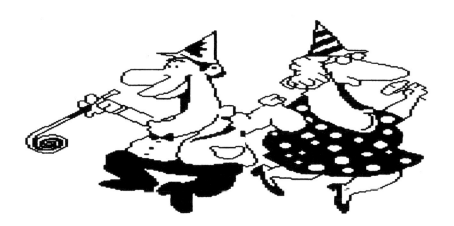

PURPOSE OF HOLIDAY SOCIALS

- To reach out to families who are reluctant to participate in other, more formal family programs
- To inform family members about other family programs being offered at the nursing home and encourage participation in these groups
- To create a relaxed atmosphere for families to get to know each other
- To provide an opportunity for the Family Council to demonstrate its leadership abilities

HELPFUL HINTS ON GETTING STARTED

Table 4.1 projects the needs of a Holiday Social and provides suggestions for creating a festive atmosphere.

TABLE 4.1. Holiday Social Characteristics

Considerations	Suggestions	Anticipated Outcome
physical setting	auditorium, lobby, or dining room in large area	promotes freedom of movement
seating arrangement	chairs (tables for food and display only)	encourages casual atmosphere
refreshments	holiday-appropriate pastries and beverages	coincides with holiday theme
# invited to social	total family population and residents	15-50 percent response
method of invitation	posters and mailed flyers with RSVP	RSVP helps to plan appropriate space/food
frequency/duration of social	2 or 3 times a year/up to 2 hours each social	allows families to "drop in"
time frame	on or close to the holiday	allows for families' varied schedules
displays	crafts, decorations, and musical entertainment	keeps holiday focus
hosts	Family Council with help of staff	promotes family participation/ownership

THE BEST TIME FOR A HOLIDAY SOCIAL

Usually the best time for a holiday get-together at the nursing home is before or after a holiday. However, if it is a holiday in honor of the residents such as Father's Day or Mother's Day, then a Holiday Social could occur on the designated holiday. Be careful of scheduling Holiday Socials the same time high school or college graduations are being held. To avoid the hustle and bustle of December, a post-holiday social in January might be of interest to a larger number of people.

INVITATIONS

Six weeks prior to the Holiday Social, the nursing home staff should send a flyer to family members. An example of a flyer is located in the Appendix. To facilitate planning for seating arrangements and refreshments, the flyer asks family members to RSVP. If there is a Family Council or group of active family members, they can help prepare the flyers to be mailed.

Usually, nursing homes have a computerized mailing list of the names and addresses of each resident's designated representative, which makes labeling envelopes to be mailed much easier. However, these mailing lists usually include only one of the resident's family members and, unfortunately, other family members may not be notified of the event. In order to extend the invitation to other family members and friends, obtain names and addresses from the guest book that is usually signed by visitors. Staff can also ask residents if they would like to invite someone other than the designated representative. In addition, posters of the Holiday Social can inform visitors of the upcoming event.

Each family member is encouraged to bring his or her resident to the Holiday Social. In fact, this is the only family program discussed in this book that residents are invited to attend.

WHAT YOU NEED TO BEGIN

A Group of People to Host the Holiday Social

If the nursing home has established a Family Council, then Council members will host the event. The nursing home will furnish the room, appropriate musical entertainment, and refreshments for the Holiday Social, but Council members will take responsibility for greeting the guests and serving refreshments. In addition, at least one of the hosts will serve as "Master of Ceremonies," or emcee. The emcee has a critical role in making certain the Holiday Social flows smoothly. Two of the responsibilities of the emcee will be to bring attention to various display tables and to announce special events occurring throughout the Social. If the nursing home has not established a Family Council, staff members will host the Holiday Social and ask family members for assistance.

Name Tags

Each family member who arrives at the Holiday Social should be greeted immediately by one of the hosts and given a name tag to wear. Name tags provide an excellent means by which family members can identify and recognize one another. For those families who notified the nursing home of their plans to attend, name tags could be prepared prior to the Social. A table can be set up for families to collect their name tags as they arrive. One of the hosts can stay at the table and assist family members in finding their name tags and also write new ones.

Another responsibility of one of the hosts is to ensure that everyone has a name tag throughout the duration of the program. Name tags may fall off, or a family member may not receive one upon arrival; therefore, another host should be specifically assigned to make sure everyone has one. Because this duty provides a reason to mingle with the crowd, it is best to assign this duty to someone who is somewhat hesitant about starting conversations. Assigning specific tasks to Family Council members promotes a smooth-flowing event, while also gives members a sense of purpose.

Displays

It is easier for people to mingle in a crowd if there is a focal point–something that everyone is looking at and talking about. Displaying the residents' latest craft or artwork during the Holiday Social provides a focal point. Whenever possible, the display should be appropriate to the holiday being celebrated. If the resident population is unable to provide anything to display, families or staff members may have items such as antiques, models of trains or cars, or stamp collections to exhibit.

Another idea for providing a focal point is to hold a pie contest. Families are encouraged to prepare their finest pie and enter it in a contest held during the Holiday Social. Contest participants are urged to involve their residents by either using the resident's recipe or having the resident help prepare the pie. Residents attending the Holiday Social, who are able to participate as impartial judges, will taste each pie and choose the first, second, and third prize-winning recipes. If residents are unable to participate in the judging aspect of the contest, perhaps impartial family or staff members can help with the decisionmaking. All of the pies can then be added to the other refreshments, or they can be used later for prizes.

An Activity

Another way to help family members meet and get to know each other is to have a planned activity. Thirty minutes into the Social, the hosts will provide everyone with a piece of paper with the following categories listed:

- Find a resident whose name begins with an "O" (or another odd letter of the alphabet)

- Find the family member who traveled the greatest distance to come to the Holiday Social
- Find a family member who has traveled overseas in the past year
- Find the resident with the most grandchildren
- Find the newest resident of the nursing home

The hosts will ask each family member to find people at the Holiday Social who fit each category. When a family member finds a person who fits one of the categories, he or she draws a check mark next to the category and writes down that person's name. Participants should be given approximately twenty minutes for this activity. The emcee announces when the activity has ended and asks family members to share their findings for each category. Finally, the emcee should ask if there are any family members who found people that fit each of the five categories. A prize could be awarded to any family member who has done so.

A Marketing Table

Attach to a table a large sign on which the following is written, "Join Us." On the table, display photographs of other family programs that were held in the past. Also make available flyers or brochures with brief descriptions of other family programs and when each program is offered. If families want to obtain information about other programs at another time, have a pile of postcards on the table that are addressed to the Family Council. See Figure 4.1 for an example. The postcards can be completed that day or mailed later to the nursing home.

To call attention to the marketing table, the emcee should announce that there is a table set up to acquaint families with other programs offered at the nursing home. In addition, the emcee should announce that a 50/50 raffle is being held to sponsor future family events and that tickets can be purchased at the table. Family members will be drawn to the table either to learn

FIGURE 4.1. Sample Postcard to Offer Information About Other Programs

Dear Family Council,

I would like to know more about:

___ **Educational Workshop**   ___ **Family Support Group**   ___ **Family Council**

My name is_____ . Please send me information at _____

_____ or call me at:_____

more about other family programs or to purchase a raffle ticket. Other prizes to raffle could include the winning pies or the crafts or artwork being displayed by the residents. The emcee should announce the winner(s) of the raffle a few minutes before the Holiday Social ends.

At the time when the winning raffle tickets are announced, the emcee should thank everyone for attending the Holiday Social. Any other announcements can be made at this time, and although the Social is officially over, the emcee should encourage people to stay and visit for as long as they wish.

This chapter described how to use social gatherings for bringing residents and their families together. In creating an informal atmosphere for families to socialize, you attract families who historically have not been interested in more official or instructional programs. In doing so, you provide yet another avenue for family involvement.

The next section expands on the programs presented in previous chapters by discussing what to do if families do not appear interested in programs or how to capitalize on the amount of interest that does exist.

Chapter 5

Lack of Family Participation and Why

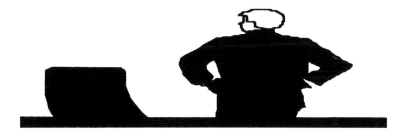

THE MYTH OF ABANDONMENT

The idea that people abandon friends and relatives once they are placed in a nursing home has been repeatedly discounted in research projects. York and Calsyn (1977) reported that families are just as involved with relatives in nursing homes as they were prior to placement. It was noted later by Bitzan and Kruzich (1990) that although families do not abandon relatives in nursing homes, the frequency of visits eventually tapers off. Perhaps the strongest evidence that this is true is our own personal experiences and disappointments in trying to engage family particiation in the nursing home.

Although this book has attempted to point nursing homes in the direction of successful family programming, reading this book does not guarantee success. People's backgrounds vary so greatly that the guidelines and suggestions offered in this book need to be tailored to the unique needs of your nursing home and family population. No one can better inform you about getting families together than your own staff and the families of your residents. If you have determined that there is a lack of interest in the family programs being offered at your nursing home, be sure the programs you are offering meet the unique needs of your residents' families.

In order to assess the interests and needs of the family population, distribute a survey. The results of the survey will indicate what programs, if any, families are interested in. The survey will also indicate what potential barriers may hinder family involvement. Sometimes it is just a matter of timing or transportation, and if you know this ahead of time, you can plan accordingly. A sample of a survey to send to families can be found in the Appendix.

Once you have held a program, it is important to find out if it would be worthwhile to offer the program again to other families. One of the best ways to determine if a program has produced its desired effect is to have families complete an evaluation at the end of the program. Samples of evaluations for each of the programs discussed in this book can be found in the Appendix. The completed evaluations will gauge the effectiveness of each program. You will find out if the program was helpful to participants and if not, what changes need to be made. A major overhaul will rarely be needed—sometimes all that needs to be improved is the room temperature.

Finally, examine the criteria used to determine whether a family program has been successful or not. Consider the following questions:

- How many family members need to express an interest in attending a program to make it worth my time and energy?
- Is there a quota or a percentage of people who must attend a program in order for it to be regarded a success?
- When staff members ask, "How many families came to the support group last night?" what reported number would gain their approval? Is that even an important question, or do staff members need a better understanding of what constitutes a successful program?

These questions need to be considered before you decide to offer family programs. Generally speaking, a program is worth pursuing if at least 15 percent of the family population express an interest. If less than 15 percent are interested, there may not be a need for that type of program, and other types of programs should be explored. If less than 15 percent express an interest in a program, you should contact these families and explain that there was not enough interest in holding that program; however, you would like to know what they hoped to get out of the program. Perhaps then a modified version could be offered to meet their needs. Holding the program without additional staff support or speakers may be an efficient alternative. On the other hand, you could keep the original format and invite other people from the community to attend. The few family members who expressed an interest in attending could be encouraged to invite friends who may be considering nursing home placement for a loved one. The program could also be brought to the attention of area hospitals and local public health agencies. These agencies could make the program known to families of patients who are in need of long-term care. Extending invitations in this manner not only helps to meet the needs of the community, but also gains public respect, which is an important part of consumer relations.

In addition to ascertaining what programs to offer at the nursing home, surveying the family population will help you to capitalize on even a small amount of interest. For example, you may discover that many families prefer to be involved only from a distance, such as by mail or telephone. In that case, much of your family programming would seek to enhance communications among families, residents, and staff members through a variety of correspondence projects. Such projects could involve:

- a facility newsletter encouraging families to submit articles or help with editing and distribution.
- telephone conferences with the interdisciplinary team to discuss resident care issues.
- a (1-800) toll-free telephone number for families who live out-of-state to maintain contact with staff.
- a library of video/audiotapes to loan families who are interested in learning more about certain topics such as "Alzheimer's and You" or "How to Make Visits Count When You Live So Far Away."

THE ROLE AND RESPONSIBILITY
OF FAMILY IN THE NURSING HOME

While some families are not "connected" to the nursing home due to geographic limitations, other families may remain distant because of psychological barriers. Many families view the nursing home as an extension of a hospital. The nursing home, like the hospital, is a place where families may think they are supposed to "stay out of the way." Families will not know anything different is expected of them at the nursing home, unless they are told.

Research concerning family involvement supports taking a direct approach with families by talking to them about their role in the nursing home. Rubin and Shuttlesworth (1983) and Schwartz and Vogel (1990) found that when staff members talked to families about what support they could and should provide at the nursing home, families were usually willing to assume a larger role.

One way of clarifying the family's role and responsibilities is to develop certain policies pertaining to family involvement. The nursing home can reasonably expect families to abide by these policies as long as they have been promptly informed of the guidelines and rules. The resident's stay at the nursing home may not necessarily be conditional upon the adherence of these rules; however, these policies convey what the nursing home expects of the family. The idea of having family members abide by rules is not a new concept. Many nursing homes already have rules established about family behavior, such as no smoking in the nursing home, checking with nursing staff before giving food or alcohol to the resident, or calling ahead of time to take a resident overnight. In this same vein, and in accordance with the residents' needs, families could be told that the nursing home requires a certain level of participation by the family.

PARTICIPATING IN CARE-PLANNING MEETINGS

Assuming the resident does not object, family members should be expected to attend care-planning meetings. A care-planning meeting is held a few days after admission and at least annually thereafter, to discuss ways to keep the resident functioning at the highest practicable level. These meetings provide one of the best forums for the interdisciplinary team and the resident's family to work together to develop a plan of care to meet the resident's needs. For example, if the interdisciplinary team makes a decision at a care-planning meeting to remove a physical restraint, and the family is not at the meeting when this change is made, the family may object, having not been part of the decision-making process. If a family member is at the care-planning meeting and can give input and ask questions about the restraint use, he or she is more likely to understand and agree with the decision.

The interdisciplinary team should do everything within its power to accommodate the family. Care-planning meetings are usually held at the same time every week so that staff members can plan their routine around the meetings. The meetings should actually be scheduled at the family's convenience. During the meetings the interdisciplinary team should make every attempt to avoid using jargon or abbreviations such as ROM (range of motion) that the family may not understand. Family members should feel encouraged to actively participate in the care-planning meeting. If a family member is quietly listening to what staff have to say about his or her resident and has nothing to add, something is wrong, and the meeting is not serving its purpose.

The team member who is facilitating should state that in developing a plan of care to meet the resident's needs, it is not the intention of the interdisciplinary team to act alone, without family input. One of the main purposes of having family at the meeting is to see the resident's problems, needs, and strengths through the family's eyes. The nursing home recognizes that it cannot always know what is best for the resident. The resident may need the specialized environment of a nursing home while also needing care that preserves or maintains his or her individuality. Providing care day after day, combined with low staffing patterns, puts care at risk of becoming mechanical and impersonal. The family members may not have the ability to provide skilled technical care, but they know enough about the resident's needs and preferences to help staff give individualized care. The family can share information with the interdisciplinary team about the resident's history, customary routines, and lifetime patterns. In this vein, the family helps staff from feeling that their work is dull and mechanical.

The interdisciplinary team often overlooks the other advantage of having family at the care-planning meeting–the family can assume some of the responsibilities listed on the care plan. Usually, ways in which the family could and should help are not discussed at care-planning meetings. Because it is assumed that the interdisciplinary team is responsible for performing all tasks outlined on the care plan, the objectives rarely include family assignments. While it is true that the nursing home is mandated by law to provide care and services to each resident, families are often willing to assume some responsibilities as long as the tasks are not too technical. In accordance with the comprehensive assessment of the resident's needs, the care plan should reflect any tasks the family has accepted or offered to perform. For example, if the family is interested in sitting with the resident at certain times of the day or week in an effort to reduce the use of a physical restraint, this assignment should be written on the care plan.

AN ORIENTATION PROGRAM

In helping to clarify the family's role in the nursing home, the family should view an orientation program on videotape. Ideally, the tape should be viewed prior to admission. However, not all admissions are planned for ahead of time, so some families would have to watch the tape on the day of admission or shortly thereafter. The videotape does not need to be more than one hour long and can be viewed at the nursing home. Important material to cover on the video tape is included in Table 5.1.

TABLE 5.1. An Orientation Program on Videotape

Personal belongings and room furnishings to bring for the resident's room
  family photographs, bedspreads, knickknacks, furniture
What is and is not included in the cost of care
  resident care equipment such as toothbrushes, hairbrushes, combs,
  linens, soap, incontinence products, medications, wheelchairs, canes,
  and cable and telephone hookups
Family Rights
  information regarding the family's right to organize a group, make health
  care decisions, contact the ombudsman and other advocating agencies
The resident assessment process
  Minimum Data Set (MDS) and care planning meetings
Tips on how to visit during the first few weeks of admission
  the first two weeks of adjustment and what to expect
Departmental policies involving family members
  family role and responsibilities in the nursing home

Rather than having one staff member talking about all the services that are provided at the nursing home, each department should explain the services it provides. Representatives from each department should introduce themselves, give a brief description of their jobs, and discuss any departmental policies they think families should know about. For example, the dietary department would explain that its job is to prepare food that is nutritious, appetizing, attractive, and served to the residents at proper temperatures. During the taped presentation, a dietary staff member could take the time to encourage families to dine with their resident and explain how to order and pay for a meal. If a family would like to hold a private party, the dietary staff member could suggest consulting the department ahead of time so that a room can be reserved and refreshments can be prepared. Any restrictions about bringing food to the resident or storing food in the room could also be discussed.

Other policies different departments need to explain on the tape include:

- procedures requiring families to call ahead of time before taking residents out overnight or for long day trips.
- how often baths are given and how frequently bed linen gets changed.
- the procedure for labeling clothes upon admission and what to do when clothes are brought in after admission.
- policies regarding family input on the use of physical restraints.

Naturally, it is important to keep the videotape current to reflect any changes in policies or staffing. If you have several new admissions in a short period of time, you may want to invite several families to view the videotape together. Staff may actually prefer to do the orientation program in person rather than on video. Although this is a more personal approach, there are some disadvantages to doing it this way. One problem with doing the program in person is that some families may not be able to attend on the date the program is scheduled. The second problem with holding an orientation program in person is that the program will not always be timely. A family member could conceivably place a relative in the nursing home four to eight weeks before the next program is offered. By the time the orientation program is offered, the information will be nonessential.

Another suggestion for an orientation program involves having a current resident's family member work with the family of a new admission. On the day of admission, have a family member who is actively involved in the nursing home, and would do an admirable job of representing the home, take the new admission's family on a tour of the facility. The tour would include introductions to key personnel and would also orient new family members to the layout and routines of the nursing home.

Arranging tours given by residents' family members is beneficial for several reasons. First, having a current resident's family member play a guiding role in the admission process gives the new family an indication of the level of family involvement that is encouraged in the nursing home. It sends a message that the facility does not want family to remain on the side-lines, but rather to actively participate in the daily operations of the nursing home. Second, putting the new family immediately in touch with another resident's family helps to create a supportive environment. Family members will find it consoling to be shown the way by another family member who has been "where they are headed." Finally, having a current resident's family member give the orientation tour is a very practical way to help the new family classify information on a "need to know" basis. The family member giving the tour has first-hand experience with the people and policies of the nursing home. The family member's perceptions are derived from experiencing the conditions in the nursing home all hours of the day—especially during evenings and on weekends. Staff members give a very different kind of tour because their perceptions are based on the shift they work and their advice comes from the viewpoint of someone who provides, not receives services. A family member will offer "insider's" information and down-to-earth advice about how to adapt to the nursing home environment.

Obviously, the family member selected to give orientation tours should be an individual who can be trusted to give a positive, but realistic view of the nursing home. Someone who had no difficulties at all adapting to the nursing home environment may not be helpful to someone who is having, or may have, a difficult adjustment period. The family member giving the tour must be familiar with both the positive and negative effects of nursing home life. Table 2.3 in Chapter 2, will help you select a family member who would be a helpful resource.

This chapter provided you with an overview of what to do when families do not seem interested in attending family programs at the nursing home. You were given practical ideas for making families aware of their role in the nursing home and the level of involvement that is expected of them. Also discussed were ways to capitalize on the amount or type of involvement families prefer to have at the nursing home.

The Appendix that follows provides you with tools that will help you to communicate with families about family programming.

Appendix

FAMILY NEEDS SURVEY

Family Programs to Offer	Check (4) That Most Interest You
General family meetings to talk about problems	
Family support group meetings to talk about feelings	
Invite families to join residents in a craft project	
Invite families to care-planning conferences	
Invite families to policy-making conferences	
Mail families educational pamphlets	
Loan educational tapes to families	
Family socials during holidays	
Send a newsletter to families	
Invite families to meet with department heads	
Orientation program for new families	
Offer a 1-800 (toll-free) number for families to use	
Hold a "Staff Appreciation Day" (sponsored by families)	
Annual brunches/picnics for residents and families	
Other . . .	
Times to Offer Programs	Check Best Times for You
Winter	
Spring	
Summer	
Fall	
Weeknight	
Weekday	
Weekend	
After supper	
Before supper	
Before dark	
Other . . .	
If programs interest you, are you likely to attend?	Circle "yes" or "no"

Reasons for Not Being Able to Attend	Check All That Apply
Transportation	
Child care	
No time	
Too far to drive	
No one to come with	
Not interested	
Don't know	
Feel awkward in nursing home	
Other . . .	
Educational Topics	Which Topics Interest You
How to Make Visits Count	
All About Alzheimer's Disease	
Communicating with Staff	
Understanding Medicare and Medicaid	
Other . . .	

FAMILY WORKSHOP INVITATION

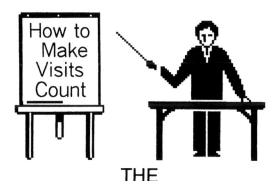

THE
NAME OF YOUR NURSING HOME
INVITES YOU AND YOUR FAMILY
TO AN EDUCATIONAL WORKSHOP
ON DATE
AT TIME

IN THE NAME OF THE ROOM
TOPICS TO BE DISCUSSED INCLUDE:
- STRESS ASSOCIATED WITH AGING
- ENHANCING STAFF/FAMILY COMMUNICATIONS
- UNDERSTANDING MEDICARE AND MEDICAID
- MAKING VISITS COUNT

---

tear here and return by   DATE   to register

YES! I AM PLANNING TO ATTEND
THE FAMILY WORKSHOP
ON DATE

NAME:_____

ATTENDING: _____

PHONE #: _____

ADDITIONAL TOPICS OF INTEREST:

STRESSORS ASSOCIATED WITH AGING

Social Stress

- *Advertisement:* marketing is ageist and aimed at staying young.
- *Stereotypes:* an older person is often viewed as forgetful, purposeless, frail, and poor.
- *Change of Status.*

Stress of Bodily Changes

- *Physical Characteristics:* skin discoloration, loss of muscle tone, loss of hair or hair pigment.
- *Sensory Organs:* loss of taste buds, smell, vision, hearing, touch.
- *Learning and Memory:* impairment, slowing down of reaction time, memory decline in retrieving words, learning deficiencies.
- *Diseases:* neurological disorders, heart and lung diseases, muscle and bone diseases.

Psychological Stress

- *Fears:* worries about maintaining independence and control.
- *Losses:* loss of companionship, a familiar standard of living, a sense of security or safety.
- *Self-Image:* changes in skin, muscle tone, and hair, identity crisis, poor self-esteem.
- *Coping Styles:* loss of lifetime coping techniques such as jogging, shopping, reading.
- *Nostalgia:* unresolved regrets and preoccupation with the past.

Financial Stress

- *Loss of Income.*
- *Health Insurance Premiums and Deductibles.*
- *Taxes.*

TIPS ON HOW TO MAKE VISITS COUNT

Conversational Ideas

- Look at the weekly calendar of activities and ask the resident if he or she went or plans to go to any of the scheduled activities. Reminisce about past-time leisure activities.
- Comment on dress or hair. Show photographs of the latest hair styles and wedding dresses. Talk about different hairstyles the resident has had.
- Refer to items in the room such as photographs or greeting cards that have arrived in the mail.
- Talk about what is happening at home with the house, family, or local church.
- Keep a logbook of whatever it is that you talk about during the visit–date and sign it. Then, if the resident has trouble remembering your visits, staff can refer to the logbook to help the resident remember.

Things to Do

- Bring a cookie mix and combine ingredients. Have the resident mix and stir if possible. Test taste from the spoon! Ask the kitchen to bake them.
- Go to one of the activities of the day.
- Watch a family video. Invite other residents.
- Stay in the resident's room and play music. Dance for, or with, the resident as able. Don't be inhibited! Be playful and lighthearted.
- Go out for a drive, dinner, or even a fast-food meal.
- Apply lotion, give a manicure or facial.
- Write a letter to friends or family.
- Bring an electric skillet and make French toast. The aroma is very stimulating.
- Bring a shoebox with nostalgic items to trigger memories such as seashells, medals of honor, sports items, cooking

utensils, car parts, replicas of farm animals, or other items related to the resident's occupation.

- Read triumphant stories from the *Reader's Digest.* (These stories can be very inspirational.)

Other Tips

- Always take at least five minutes prior to coming to the nursing home to think about conversational ideas and things to do. Use physical props whenever possible.
- Plan for periods of silence. Tell yourself that you can handle five or ten minutes of nothing but silence. Show the resident you are quite comfortable with silence.
- When visiting a resident with dementia, accept his or her input, no matter how irrelevant it might be. Even an irrelevant comment is an attempt to be part of the conversation. If a disoriented resident is preoccupied with finding someone or something that no longer exists, ask who, what, and where questions that help the resident play out his or her fantasy.

Resident: Can you help me find my mother?
   Visitor: When was the last time you saw her?
            Where might she be at this time of day?
            What is it that you're missing about your mother?

You don't always have to enforce the truth:

Resident: Can you help me find my mother?
   Visitor: She died; don't you remember?

Try distraction:

Visitor: I can't help you with that but did I tell you I'm going to can tomatoes tomorrow?
            Do you remember canning tomatoes? How did you do it?

Listen for the meaning or feeling behind the words. Words are a very small part of communication. Use more body language than any other kind of communication.

- If you are visiting a resident who constantly complains remember that it is just his or her way of letting you know he or she is still hanging in there. Complaints are better than silence and withdrawal. You do not always have to fix whatever is wrong. Sometimes it is important to just listen and validate the resident's feeling. However, sometimes it may be necessary to tell the resident that you would rather talk about something else and if that is not possible you will have to leave.
- Let the staff members know how your visit went. This gives you an opportunity to get to know staff members and for them to support your involvement. This is important especially in situations where the resident did not appear to respond to your visit. The staff members like the opportunity to reassure you that even though the resident did not seem to recognize you, the resident still needs to be nurtured with love and attention. The resident's identity is preserved when the resident is being respected and honored by the family.

PROGRAM EVALUATIONS

I. Educational Family Workshop Evaluation

Please complete the following statements by checking the column that best describes your rating:

Characteristics	Excellent	Good	Fair	Poor
Personal needs met				
Value of meeting and talking with staff				
Speaker's manner of organization				
Information and knowledge presented				
Physical setting of the room				
Being with other families				
Likelihood of attending other programs				
Overall rating of the Family Workshop				

Additional Comments:

II. Family Support Group Evaluation

Please complete the following statements by checking the
column that best describes your rating:

Characteristics	Excellent	Good	Fair	Poor
Personal needs met				
Value of being with other families				
Physical setting of the room				
Supportive atmosphere of the group				
Opportunities for sharing my experiences				
Opportunities for helping others				
Refreshments				
Overall rating of the support group				

Additional Comments:

III. Family Council Evaluation

Please complete the following statements by checking the column that best describes your rating:

Characteristics	Excellent	Good	Fair	Poor
Family Council makes a difference				
Value of being with other families				
Value of meeting and talking with staff				
Opportunity to positively affect the nursing home				
Opportunity to have input in decisions				
Physical setting of the room				
Overall rating of the Family Council				

Additional Comments:

IV. Holiday Social Evaluation

Please complete the following statements by checking the column that best describes your rating:

Characteristics	Excellent	Good	Fair	Poor
Value of celebrating the holiday with my resident				
Value of meeting and talking with other families				
Opportunity to meet other residents				
Atmosphere of the Social				
Personal needs met				
Physical setting of the room				
Overall rating of the Holiday Social				

Additional Comments:

FAMILY SUPPORT GROUP INVITATION

(Front)

Having a loved one in a nursing home isn't easy...

...so we turn to others for help

(Inside)

You are invited to a Family Support Group meeting held every _____ at _____ at the _____ in _____

Hope you can join us.

FAMILY SOCIAL INVITATIONS

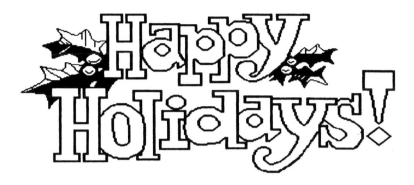

THE FAMILY COUNCIL, RESIDENTS, AND STAFF OF THE

REQUEST THE PLEASURE OF YOUR COMPANY FOR *POST*HOLIDAY REFRESHMENTS ON SUNDAY, THE   OF JANUARY 2:30 PM UNTIL 3:30 PM

---

tear here and return by   to register

YES! I AM PLANNING TO ATTEND *THE POSTHOLIDAY SOCIAL*
NAME:_____

RESIDENT:_____

ATTENDING: _____

PHONE #:_____

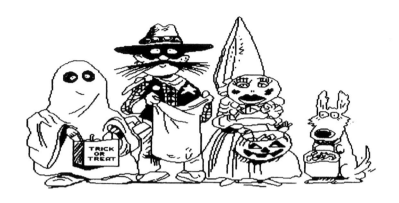

THE FAMILY COUNCIL
OF THE
INUITES YOU AND YOUR RESIDENT
FOR DOUGHNUTS AND CIDER
ON
AT
PLEASE LET US KNOW IF YOU CAN ATTEND

tear here and return by   to register

YES! I AM PLANNING TO ATTEND
THE HOLIDAY SOCIAL
NAME:_____

RESIDENT:_____

ATTENDING: _____

PHONE #: _____

References

Bitzan, Janet E. and Jean M. Kruzich. (1990). Interpersonal relationships of nursing home residents. *The Gerontologist*, 30, 385-390.

Rubin, Allen and Guy Shuttlesworth. (1983). Engaging families as support resources in nursing home care: Ambiguity in the subdivision of tasks. *The Gerontologist*, 23, 632-636.

Schwartz, Arthur N. and Mark Vogel. (1990). Nursing home staff and residents' families role expectations. *The Gerontologist*, 30, 49-53.

York, Jonathan L. and Robert Calsyn. (1977). Family involvement in nursing homes. *The Gerontologist*, 17, 500-505.

Index

Page numbers in italics refer to tables, charts, or material found in the appendix.